1200 MCQs in Medicine

Co-authors

J. Anderson

MB, BS, FRCP,
Academic Sub-Dean, The Medical School,
Senior Lecturer in Medicine, The University
of Newcastle upon Tyne; Honorary Consultant
Physician, The Royal Victoria Infirmary,
Newcastle

E.B. French

MB, BChir, FRCP,
Lately Physician to the Northern Group
of Hospitals, Edinburgh

P.H. Sanderson

MB, BChir, FRCP,
Consulting Physician, St. Mary's Hospital,
London

C.C. Smith

MB, Ed., FRCP,
Consultant Physician, The City Hospital,
Aberdeen; Honorary Senior Lecturer in
Medicine, Department of Medicine, The
University of Aberdeen, Aberdeen

J.F. Stokes

MD, FRCP, FRCP (Ed.),
Consulting Physician, University
College Hospital, London

1200 MCQs in Medicine

A supplement to
Macleod's CLINICAL EXAMINATION and
DAVIDSON'S PRINCIPLES AND PRACTICE OF MEDICINE

Edited by

P.R. Fleming

MD, FRCP, DHMSA,
Senior Lecturer in Medicine,
Westminster Medical School;
Consultant Physician, Westminster Hospital,
London

Foreword by J.G. Macleod

MB, ChB, FRCP (Ed.),
Lately Chairman of University Department
of Medicine, Western General Infirmary,
Edinburgh

CHURCHILL LIVINGSTONE
EDINBURGH LONDON AND NEW YORK 1980

CHURCHILL LIVINGSTONE
Medical Division of Longman Group Limited

Distributed in the United States of America by
Churchill Livingstone Inc., 1560 Broadway,
New York, N.Y. 10036, and by associated
companies, branches and representatives
throughout the world.

First published 1980
Reprinted 1981
Reprinted 1983
Reprinted 1984

ISBN 0 443 01571 6

British Library Cataloguing in Publication Data

1200 MCQs in medicine.
    1. Pathology — Examinations, questions, etc.
    I. Fleming, Peter Robert II. Macleod, John, *b. 1915*.
    Clinical examination III. Davidson, *Sir* Stanley.
    Davidson's principles and practice of medicine
    IV. Thousand two hundred MCQs in medicine
    616'. 007'6   RB119   79-42808

Printed in Hong Kong by Sing Cheong Printing Co Ltd

Foreword

The study of textbooks, and teaching by question and answer along time-honoured Socratic lines, continue to provide the main methods of learning for most of us, with audio-visual aids giving further refinement more recently. I therefore welcomed the suggestion made by Dr Fleming and his colleagues that *Davidson's Principles and Practice of Medicine* and *Clinical Examination,* both of which I edit, should be supplemented by the publication of a book of multiple choice questions.

Well constructed MCQs are internationally accepted as an efficient method for the assessment of knowledge and can be used for this purpose both by examining bodies and by individuals; for the latter they also provide a valuable adjunct to learning. Furthermore I visualised receiving constructive feedback from the authors which would benefit the parent textbooks. My expectations have been met fully in all regards. Dr Fleming and his team, with much expertise and care, have produced a wide range of questions specifically designed to test the knowledge and skills of the reader in regard to the fundamentals of the practice of medicine.

Edinburgh, 1980   J. MacL

Preface

Most parents will be familiar with requests from their children to 'hear my homework' and will have felt obliged to listen, book in hand, to a stumbling recitation of *The Charge of the Light Brigade* or a list of French irregular verbs. Tedious as this exercise undoubtedly is, the child's request is, nevertheless, based upon the sound principle that assessment immediately after a period of learning consolidates the knowledge acquired and allows both teachers and taught to proceed to their next task with confidence.

It is upon this principle that the multiple-choice questions in this book have been prepared; its purpose is to allow those who read the two standard textbooks on which it is based—*Davidson's Principles and Practice of Medicine* and Macleod's *Clinical Examination*—to determine whether they have retained the information acquired in their reading and, if this is not the case, to point clearly to the areas in which revision is required. The questions contain material which is all dealt with in either 'Davidson' or 'Macleod' and they can be answered either by direct reference to statements in those books or, occasionally, by a reasonable inference from such statements. The authors confess to having been tempted, from time to time, to include items which were not referred to in the texts but they are confident that they have successfully resisted this temptation and believe that, had they not done so, much of the value of this book would have been lost.

Most of the questions are arranged according to the corresponding chapters of 'Davidson' or 'Macleod' and refer to material all of which can be found in the appropriate chapter; they can, therefore, be attempted immediately after that chapter has been read. All of the questions in this section are of the Independent True/False type. The questions which are not arranged in this way include some which refer to more than one chapter of either of the books; many are in the Independent True/False format but some are of the One-from-Five type and others are in the format known as Relationship Analysis in which knowledge of factual statements and of the causal relationships between them is tested.

The authors are well aware of the need to avoid ambiguity in multiple-choice questions and, having had a fair amount of experience in this area, have applied the usual rules in their construction. In some cases, however, it has been possible, by virtue of the close correspondence between the questions and the statements in the textbooks to which they refer, to avoid the somewhat stilted English which may be necessary to render multiple-choice questions completely clear and unambiguous.

No one, least of all the authors of this book, would suggest that facility in answering multiple-choice questions guarantees sufficient knowledge, in the widest sense, for the practice of medicine. The manipulation of information needed for the understanding of pathophysiological processes and the solution of diagnostic and therapeutic problems can rarely be tested thoroughly by the multiple-choice technique; the modest aim of this book is to help students increase the efficiency with which they acquire the factual knowledge on which medical practice is based.

London, 1980   P.R.F.

Advice to readers

The questions in this book have been set primarily as an aid to learning although they will, of course, be useful to those who are preparing specifically for an examination in which MCQs play a part. To use them to their best advantage you should read a chapter in one of the textbooks and then attempt the appropriate questions. Reference to the Answer Key will allow you to check your accuracy and where you find that you have incorrectly identified an item as True or False you should immediately refer back to the original text to see how your error has arisen. The discipline of immediately searching for information is advocated not on account of a puritanical idea that hard work is good for everyone but because the authors believe that this is an efficient way of acquiring and retaining information.

The questions in Part Two are not arranged under chapter numbers (although they do run in parallel with the texts) and are designed for general revision. In this part you should pay special attention to the different question formats used and, in particular, must not confuse the questions of the Independent True/False type with those in the One-from-Five format. If you wish to use this part as a trial examination paper, two hours would be a reasonable period of time to allow yourself for its completion.

Contents

Contents

PART ONE

In this part the questions are of the Independent True/False type. Any number of items, or all or none of them, may be correct. The questions are arranged according to the chapters of (1) Macleod's *Clinical Examination* (Questions 1-250) and (2) Davidson's *Principles and Practice of Medicine* (Questions 251-1100).

Section 1
MCQ on Macleod's *Clinical Examination*

CHAPTER ONE

1
During the interrogation of a patient
A a history of joint pains may be suppressed if there is a family history of rheumatoid arthritis
B it is important to put leading questions early to the elderly
C his account should be kept to essentials by frequent tactful interruptions
D vague terms such as 'indigestion' should be avoided in the systemic enquiry
E it is important to remember that he may have been deliberately misled by his previous doctors

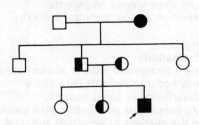

2
From the pedigree chart above the following conclusions can be drawn:
A The patient in whom the disease was observed was a male
B The patient's parents were heterozygotic for the disease
C The patient's uncle and aunt were normal
D The patient's maternal grandfather was normal
E The patient's paternal grandmother had the disease

3
Detailed enquiry about a patient's present and past occupations is important because
A he may have to be advised to change his job
B it is advisable to divert his attention from his symptoms from time to time
C frequent change of employment may indicate an inadequate personality
D some diseases may be directly due to his occupation
E advice on rehabilitation may be modified by his leisure pursuits

4
During a consultation
A it may be helpful for the clinician to make a dispassionate appraisal of the effect the patient has on him
B a clinician who receives an apparently sexual invitation from a patient should immediately transfer that patient to the care of a colleague
C the distress of a hysterical patient may be masked by apparent unconcern
D a patient's emotional problems should be discussed in the presence of a third person
E note-taking by the clinician may have an inhibiting effect on the patient when personal matters are being discussed

5
It is particularly helpful to obtain information from a third party if the patient is believed to be suffering from
A epilepsy
B diabetes mellitus
C anorexia nervosa
D deficiency of vitamin C
E dementia

6
During a physical examination
A the sequence of the examination should be the same as that in which the findings will be recorded
B observer errors are likely to occur except in the simplest observations such as localisation of the apex beat
C the patient should be in a semi-reclining position throughout
D it is wise to record the blood pressure towards the end of the examination
E it may sometimes be advisable to start the examination at a point remote from the site of the patient's complaint

7
The following statements are correct:
A When a patient is found to be hypersensitive to a drug, the fact should be recorded prominently on the front of the case notes
B A single diagnosis can nearly always explain a patient's symptoms and signs
C An attempt should be made to make a provisional diagnosis as early as possible in the clinical examination
D In most circumstances case notes should be brief and record the positive findings only
E The majority of patients dislike talking to students, however sympathetic they are

CHAPTER TWO

8
During a psychiatric interview the clinician should
A encourage the patient with expressions of sympathy or approval as seems appropriate
B allow the patient to tell his own story even if it seems that he is following a 'blind alley'
C never convey moral censure
D make a note of his own questions as well as of the patient's answers
E avoid asking the patient about suicide intentions until he is sure the patient is not depressed

9
Retardation of social growth and identity-formation in the late teens may be manifested by
A difficulty in deciding on a career
B fears about homosexuality
C formation of a close relationship with a person of the opposite sex
D over-dependence on parents
E rebellion against parental authority

10
Hallucinations
A are a recognised feature of alcoholism
B only occur in patients with some disturbance of consciousness
C are sensations perceived by the patient in the absence of an actual stimulus
D in a solitary aloof patient suggest that he has a personality disorder
E imply that the causative psychiatric disorder is irreversible

11
A patient should be suspected of having an intellectual defect if
A his speech shows lack of the expected connection between phrases
B he is unable to say where he is
C he cannot remember what he had for breakfast
D he cannot do simple arithmetic
E he displays unwarranted optimism and elation

12
One should suspect a patient of having a schizoid personality if he
A habitually exaggerates
B is very emotional
C shows a craving for attention
D is very shy
E is easily upset by disturbance of his routine

13
The following statements about psychoneurosis are correct:
A Insight is impaired
B The patient may be morbidly sorrowful to the extent of depressing the clinician also
C The patient may complain of somatic symptoms
D The patient may be helped by the communication of his experiences to the doctor
E The illness typically 'comes out of the blue'

CHAPTER THREE

14
Pain-producing substances which have been identified experimentally include
A histamine
B adrenaline
C acetyl-choline
D calcium ions
E hypertonic saline

15
Abdominal pain may arise from
A the skin when it is tightly stretched over massive ascites
B ischaemic bowel
C the congested parenchyma of the liver in acute cardiac failure
D acute distension of the splenic capsule
E spasm of the ureter

16
The pain of peptic ulcer
A is well localised in the epigastrium
B may occasionally be referred to the right shoulder tip
C is usually said to have a 'heavy' or 'crushing' quality
D is made worse by bending forwards
E is relieved by alkalis in half to one hour

17
The pain of myocardial ischaemia
A can usually be differentiated from retrosternal pain due to other lesions by its character
B is regularly induced by exercise
C may be felt in the lower jaw and tongue only
D does not usually last for more than a few seconds
E characteristically occurs in attacks with pain-free intervals lasting weeks or months

18

Typically, headaches due to

A psychological causes are felt over the frontal and occipital regions

B migraine are preceded by visual disturbances

C hypertension are often present on waking

D frontal sinusitis are worst in the evening

E migraine occur at regular and predictable times

19

Syncope

A on exertion could well be due to aortic stenosis

B on standing up could well be due to vertebro-basilar arterial disease

C following movements of the head could well be due to a hypersensitive carotid sinus reflex

D followed by a facial flush is probably an Adams-Stokes attack

E in a recumbent patient is very unlikely to be a vasovagal attack

20

Loss of consciousness with little or no warning could be

A a vasovagal attack

B an Adams-Stokes attack

C grand mal

D temporal lobe epilepsy

E cataplexy

21

Recognised features of temporal lobe epilepsy include

A prodromal flashes of light

B the 'déjà vu' phenomenon

C hallucinations of smell

D involuntary movements involving one limb

E automatism

22

Recognised causes of epilepsy include

A intracranial tumour

B renal failure

C a prolonged paroxysm of coughing

D excessive consumption of LSD

E hypoglycaemia

23

Decreased pulmonary compliance is the main cause of dyspnoea in

A left ventricular failure

B massive pulmonary embolism

C emphysema

D myasthenia gravis

E extensive pulmonary consolidation

24

In a patient suffering from paroxysmal nocturnal dyspnoea, the following signs would favour asthma rather than left ventricular failure:

A basal crepitations

B raised jugular venous pressure

C expiratory rhonchi in the absence of other signs

D central cyanosis early in the attack

E hypotension

25

Likely causes of an acute attack of dyspnoea associated with chest pain include

A spontaneous pneumothorax

B myocardial infarction

C massive intrapleural haemorrhage

D bronchial asthma

E massive pulmonary embolism

26

It is probable that a subcutaneous mass is malignant if it

A is fixed to the skin

B has a clearly defined edge

C is 'stony' hard

D is tender on palpation

E is pulsatile

27

The following statements are correct:

A Brown pigmentation in the skin over a swelling is suggestive of an aneurysm

B The pain due to erosion of bone by a tumour is often worst at night

C A friction rub may be heard over a large thyroid

D A cystic swelling is likely to show transillumination

E The surface of a simple goitre is usually smooth

28
A raised protein concentration in the interstitial fluid is an important factor in the genesis of the oedema of
A acute glomerulonephritis
B angio-oedema
C nephrotic syndrome
D kwashiorkor
E congenital lymphangiectasis

29
The hydrostatic pressure
A is much higher in the glomerular than in the pulmonary capillaries
B at the venous end of a capillary is higher than that at the arterial end
C in the capillaries of the face exceeds the plasma oncotic pressure when the subject is recumbent
D in the capillaries of the feet rises in hot weather
E is higher than normal in the capillaries of a limb of which the lymphatic drainage is blocked

30
Oedema due to hypoproteinaemia results from
A cirrhosis of the liver
B chronic pancreatitis
C acute glomerulonephritis
D repeated paracentesis of the abdomen
E nephrotic syndrome

31
Pitting oedema
A may not be clinically detectable until the extra-cellular fluid volume has increased by 10 per cent or more
B develops more quickly in a paralysed limb of the bedridden patient than in his normal limbs
C in cardiac failure is mainly due to the rise in venous pressure
D develops in all normal subjects from time to time
E is a characteristic feature of myxoedema

CHAPTER FOUR

32
During a consultation a doctor should
A refrain from making observations of the patient's demeanour until he has taken a full history
B match his attitude to that of the patient
C remember that general inspection is less important in the examination of an infant than in that of an adult
D be prepared to modify the routine of his examination according to the circumstances of the case
E pay particular attention to the patient's posture in bed

33
The complexion of a patient
A should be assessed in daylight
B may be affected by dietary habit
C is independent of the tone in the vessels of the subpapillary venous plexuses
D is a reliable guide to the presence of anaemia
E may alter as a result of chronic renal failure

34
Melanin pigmentation of the skin
A may be patchily reduced in auto-immune disease
B can be absent as a result of a genetically determined enzyme defect
C is typically reduced in amount in pregnancy
D is less obvious in scars than in normal skin in Addison's disease
E is increased in haemochromatosis

35
Involuntary movements of the hands may occur in the absence of organic disease of the central nervous system as a consequence of
A renal failure
B respiratory failure
C hepatic failure
D hypothyroidism
E chronic alcoholism

36
Halitosis
A is usually recognised by the patient before anyone else
B may be caused by atrophic rhinitis
C contrary to popular belief, is not associated with gingivitis
D has a particularly offensive odour in a case of gastrocolic fistula
E can always be explained if sufficient care is taken

37
Loss of appetite is an important cause of weight loss in
A anxiety
B diabetes mellitus
C progressive lipodystrophy
D thyrotoxicosis
E gastric carcinoma

38
Dehydration
A is easily overlooked
B is best assessed by looking at the tongue
C will not cause lowering of the blood pressure in an adult until about five litres of fluid have been lost
D can be inferred from packed cell volume even if the patient's previous state of health is unknown
E rarely affects the patient's weight

39
When taking a patient's temperature, it should be remembered that
A rectal temperature is about one degree lower than axillary temperature
B rectal readings are more reliable than recordings from the mouth
C an increased oral temperature may follow a hot bath
D feeling the patient's skin provides quite a reliable indication of fever if the thermometer is not available
E the ordinary clinical thermometer does not read below 35°C

40
Loss of scalp hair is a recognised feature of
A fungus infection
B hypogonadism
C hypopituitarism
D myotonic dystrophy
E hepatic cirrhosis

41
Swelling of the eyelids is a recognised feature of
A meningitis
B acute glomerulonephritis
C hyperthyroidism
D trichinosis
E glaucoma

42
Painful inflamed cracks at the corners of the mouth (angular stomatitis) may be due to
A infection with *Candida albicans*
B epithelioma
C the use of lipstick to which the patient is hypersensitive
D iron deficiency
E riboflavin deficiency

43
Abnormalities of the gums may be seen in patients with
A scurvy
B epilepsy under treatment
C amyloidosis
D acromegaly
E chronic lead poisoning

44
The following statements about the tongue are correct:
A Failure of protrusion may be due to modesty in the absence of organic disease
B Central cyanosis is better assessed by inspecting the tongue than the fingertips
C A geographical tongue is due to Vitamin B deficiency
D Leukoplakia is a less significant finding than excessive furring
E Patients, observing their own circumvallate papillae, may believe they have cancer of the tongue

45
Aphthous ulcers of the mouth
A are painless
B occur in crops
C are usually due to a spirochaete which can be seen on examination of a smear
D never leave a scar when healed
E often occur in patients with ulcerative colitis

46
Ulceration of the buccal mucosa is a recognised feature of
A measles
B chicken pox
C secondary syphilis
D haemochromatosis
E agranulocytosis

47
When examining the thyroid
A moderate flexion of the neck facilitates palpation of the gland from in front
B tenderness of a goitre suggests the possibility of thyroiditis
C immobility of the gland is only suggestive of carcinoma if the goitre is very large
D a bruit over the gland usually implies hyperthyroidism
E x-rays are unlikely to add to the clinical findings unless stridor is present

48
When the presence of a carcinoma of the breast is suspected
A the patient should be lying flat on a couch throughout the examination
B it is easier to see 'tethering' of the skin if the breast is gently elevated by hand
C palpation with the flat of the hand reduces the diffuse nodularity of fibrocystic disease
D examination of the axilla is of little importance once a lump in the breast has been discovered
E biopsy should rarely be needed if clinical examination is sufficiently thorough

49
Excessive sweating occurs in patients with
A cystic fibrosis
B acute hypoglycaemia
C Horner's syndrome
D hyperthyroidism
E severe pain

50
Findings which may lead towards a precise dermatological diagnosis include
A a history of having purchased a new wristwatch
B a history of contact with animals
C the presence of scratch marks
D a dry surface with bleeding points after removal of the epidermis
E the presence of genital lesions

51
Vesicular or bullous skin lesions are caused by
A herpes simplex
B herpes zoster
C barbiturate poisoning
D scabies
E Phthyrius pubis (crab louse) infestation

52
Erythema nodosum
A gives rise to painful lesions on the legs
B is associated with scleroderma
C is a recognised feature of sarcoidosis in the adult
D may be produced by sulphonamides
E may be confused with dermatitis artefacta

53
The following statements about primary skin disorders are correct:
A Psoriasis may involve the joints
B The skin cannot be moved over a sebaceous cyst
C Neurofibromas are usually associated with scattered patches of brown pigmentation
D Melanomas are only pigmented when they are very malignant
E The port wine stain type of angioma may lose its colour

54
Recognised features of heroin addiction include
A thrombosed veins
B hepatitis
C dilated pupils
D a tendency to feign illness
E tremor on withdrawal of the drug

CHAPTER FIVE

55
In a patient with known heart disease
A the three cardinal manifestations to be sought are pain, dyspnoea and oedema
B the history contributes principally to the making of the anatomical diagnosis
C an absence of symptoms excludes serious disease
D dyspnoea on effort is unequivocal evidence of cardiac failure
E a history of momentary jabs of pain at the cardiac apex is unrelated to the cardiac lesion

56
Cardiovascular conditions which may lead to acute pulmonary oedema include
A tricuspid incompetence
B myocardial infarction
C left atrial myxoma
D massive pulmonary embolism
E aortic stenosis

57
The pain of angina pectoris is characteristically
A felt maximally over the left chest
B stabbing in quality
C aggravated by hot weather
D relieved in 2–3 seconds by rest
E accompanied by dyspnoea

58
In cardiovascular disease a possible cause of
A jaundice is impairment of hepatic function
B brassy cough is tracheal compression by a hypertrophied right ventricle
C oedema is a fall in renal blood flow
D impairment of vision is a persistently high jugular venous pressure
E pain in the back is massive left atrial enlargement

59
The family, social and previous medical history are important in the diagnosis of heart disease because
A rheumatic heart disease tends to occur in families
B Marfan's syndrome is associated with cardiomyopathy
C ischaemic heart disease results from excessive consumption of alcohol
D diphtheria is frequently followed by valvular disease
E recurrent urinary infections may lead to arterial hypertension

60
The following statements are correct:
A Warm hands in an elderly female with cardiac failure are suggestive of hyperthyroidism
B If the hands, ears and cheeks are cyanosed, then a low arterial oxygen saturation can be presumed
C Clubbing of the fingers commonly accompanies large right to left shunts
D Cyanosis is a characteristic feature of left to right shunts
E A prominent arterial pulse beneath the sternal insertion of the right sternomastoid in a woman aged 55 should suggest coarctation of the aorta

61
Regarding the arterial pulse and pulse rate
A the pulse at the wrist is due to the flow of blood through the artery
B the radial pulse is synchronous with the first heart sound
C hardening and tortuosity of the radial artery is an indication of atheroma elsewhere
D sinus bradycardia may result from a rising intracranial pressure
E pressure on the carotid sinus may reduce the rate in atrial flutter

62
Pulse volume
A is best judged by determining the amount of finger pressure needed to abolish the pulse
B is proportional to local blood flow
C varies from beat to beat in ventricular tachycardia if the atria are contracting independently
D varies from beat to beat whenever the pulse is irregular
E is unaffected in constrictive pericarditis

63
Each characteristic pulse is matched against the appropriate cause for it
A alternans—extrasystoles every alternate beat
B paradoxus—pericardial effusion
C bigeminus—left bundle branch block
D collapsing—severe anaemia
E bisferiens—combined aortic stenosis and incompetence

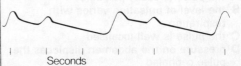

Seconds

64
The pulse illustrated above was felt in a patient with sino-atrial rate of 60/min. This finding is compatible with
A alternate atrial ectopic beats
B alternate ventricular ectopic beats
C every third beat originating from an atrial ectopic focus
D every third beat originating from a ventricular ectopic focus
E 3 : 2 heart block

65
Korotkow sounds may be heard without the application of a pressure cuff
A over the femoral artery in external iliac artery stenosis
B over an A–V fistula
C in some normal persons
D with hyperextension at the elbow
E as a result of pressing too hard with the bell of the stethoscope

66
In examining the vasomotor reflexes it is recognised that

A a fall in blood pressure in the erect position and profound bradycardia after the straining period in a Valsalva manoeuvre are likely to have the same cause

B pressure on either carotid sinus may cause syncope

C the Valsalva manoeuvre involves a strong inspiratory effort against a closed glottis

D The Valsalva manoeuvre does not affect the rate of the failing heart

E a change in intrathoracic pressure causes an equal but opposite *immediate* change in the arterial blood pressure

67
Pulsation in the neck is probably venous if

A the pulse is easily palpable

B the level of pulsation varies with respiration

C the pulse is well localised

D pressure on the abdomen displaces the pulse cephalad

E the site of pulsation in the neck is unaltered by changes in posture

68
In the jugular venous pulse

A the 'a' wave may be of unusually large amplitude when there is a left parasternal heave

B the peak of the normal 'v' wave is in mid-systole

C the 'v' wave is enhanced and earlier in onset in tricuspid regurgitation

D cannon waves are due to atrial contraction against a closed tricuspid valve

E a transient deep 'y' descent is followed by a plateau of elevated pressure in constrictive pericarditis

69
The venous pressure

A should be measured by inspection of the external jugular veins

B is recorded as the vertical height above the suprasternal notch of the uppermost venous pulse

C unlike arterial pressure, is unaffected by anxiety

D normally rises during inspiration

E is elevated early in the development of right heart failure

70
The cardiac apical impulse

A is caused by the sudden enlargement of the ventricles due to atrial contraction

B varies in position with changes in the patient's posture

C has a tapping quality in right ventricular hypertrophy

D is often impalpable in patients with emphysema

E is normally between the mid-clavicular and anterior axillary lines

71
On palpation of the praecordium

A the thrill of aortic stenosis is more easily felt on full inspiration

B a thrill may be felt even when the associated murmur is soft

C massive enlargement of the left atrium may produce an impulse to the right of the sternum

D an aortic aneurysm may produce an impulse to the right of the upper sternum

E heart sounds as well as murmurs may be felt

72
The following statements about auscultation of the heart are correct:
A The third sound immediately follows the opening of the atrioventricular valves.
B If there is an easily palpable pre-systolic impulse at the apex a loud fourth sound will certainly be heard
C A long interval between the second sound and the opening snap suggests severe mitral stenosis
D A loud opening snap suggests a calcified mitral valve
E The aortic area is the surface marking of the aortic valve

73
Light pressure with the bell of the stethoscope is required when listening for
A splitting of the second sound
B the third sound
C an opening snap
D the fourth sound
E a mitral diastolic murmur

74
The first heart sound
A is best heard at the apex of the heart
B may be louder than usual if the ecg shows a short P–R interval
C is characteristically sharp and loud in mitral regurgitation
D is closely followed by an ejection sound in aortic valve stenosis
E is louder than usual in systemic hypertension

75
A third heart sound is a recognised finding in
A mitral regurgitation
B constrictive pericarditis
C mitral stenosis
D normal children
E pulmonary stenosis

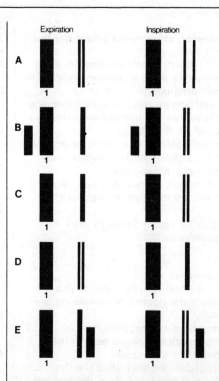

76
The following captions to the heart sound diagrams above are correct (murmurs, if any, are not shown):
A Right bundle branch block
B Systemic hypertension
C Left bundle branch block
D Pulmonary stenosis
E Left ventricular failure

77
The following statements about cardiac murmurs are correct:
A A soft early diastolic murmur in the pulmonary area is a common feature of normal pregnancy
B The ejection murmur of aortic stenosis may diminish in intensity with the onset of cardiac failure
C A mitral diastolic murmur is best heard with the patient sitting forward and breath held in expiration
D The murmurs of tricuspid and mitral stenosis are identical except for their site
E Ventricular septal defect causes a pansystolic murmur

78
The murmur of
A mitral stenosis is restricted to pre-systole if the degree of narrowing is severe
B rheumatic aortic regurgitation is characteristically heard best in the second right interspace
C aortic stenosis starts after the first sound and finishes before the second
D mitral regurgitation is conducted from the apex to the axilla and left side of the back
E patent ductus arteriosus is maximal in early systole

79
The following statements about arteries and their disorders are correct:
A The femoral may be ligated without ill effects in a healthy young person
B Pain in a severely ischaemic foot is eased by elevation of the leg
C Absence of palpable foot pulses in the elderly is a serious prognostic sign
D The contribution to the blood flow to the hand by the radial and ulnar arteries can be compared clinically
E Raynaud's disease usually implies partial occlusion of the subclavian or brachial artery

80
The following statements about veins and their disorders are correct:
A Visible veins around the umbilicus may result from portal venous obstruction
B Malaise, fever and tachycardia may signify the development of a venous thrombosis
C Trendelenberg's test assesses the competence of the venous valves in the legs
D Venous thrombosis in the legs is present in half of all patients dying in hospital
E Thrombosis of the inferior vena cava is incompatible with life

81
In the investigation of heart disease
A a PA radiograph is the best method of diagnosing right ventricular enlargement
B pulmonary arterial hypertension may produce characteristic radiographic changes
C calcification of mitral and aortic valves can be most easily identified on a PA radiograph
D echocardiography is of value in suspected mitral valve disease
E echocardiography is seldom of use in the diagnosis of a pericardial effusion

82
In cardiac failure
A acute pulmonary oedema is a characteristic complication of pulmonary arterial hypertension
B inability to lie flat in comfort is a characteristic feature of severe right heart failure
C a pleural effusion does not occur in the absence of inflammatory disease of the pleura
D in infants hepatomegaly may be a better sign than jugular venous distension
E the consequent disturbance in renal function results in the production of urine of low specific gravity

83
Features of cor pulmonale resulting from long standing emphysema include
A mental confusion
B a low arterial oxygen saturation
C coldness of the extremities
D a large 'a' wave in the jugular venous pulse
E an increased area of dullness to percussion over the heart

84
In an attack of tachycardia
A the ventricular rate is usually above 180/min if the focus is supraventricular
B the intensity of the first heart sound varies from beat to beat in ventricular tachycardia with atrio-ventricular dissociation
C a fast, irregular pulse is most likely to be due to atrial flutter with varying block
D a supraventricular origin is likely in a young patient without other evidence of heart disease
E ecg evidence of a ventricular origin is an urgent indication for digoxin treatment

85
Infective endocarditis
A is readily overlooked in elderly patients
B is easier to diagnose if it arises on a bicuspid aortic valve than on a ventricular septal defect
C causes both proteinuria and microscopic haematuria
D causes massive splenic enlargement
E may present as an obscure anaemia

CHAPTER SIX

86
In an acute respiratory illness
A pleural pain precedes pyrexia by a day or two in pneumococcal pneumonia
B cough occurs early in viral pneumonia
C failure to respond to antibiotic treatment supports the possibility of a pulmonary infarct
D it may be advisable to defer obtaining a history until dyspnoea has been relieved
E physical signs alone give a reliable indication of pulmonary tuberculosis

87
Cough may be produced by stimuli arising in the
A nasal sinuses
B main bronchi
C pulmonary alveoli
D parietal pleura
E pharynx

88
Pain is typically associated with cough in
A chronic asthma
B chronic bronchitis
C acute laryngitis
D lobar pneumonia
E tracheitis

89
The cough of chronic bronchitis characteristically
A wakes the patient in the middle of the night
B is aggravated by changes in posture
C can cause syncope
D aggravates dyspnoea
E is productive of purulent sputum

90
Sputum
A is usually saliva if the patient denies cough
B of watery consistency is characteristic of status asthmaticus
C described by the patient as 'black' indicates infection in the bronchial tree
D which is foul-smelling suggests lung abscess
E which is tenacious and rusty-coloured is characteristic of pneumococcal pneumonia.

91
Frank haemoptysis, in which the material coughed up consists wholly of blood, is to be expected in
A chronic bronchitis
B pulmonary infarction
C aortic stenosis
D bronchiectasis
E pulmonary tuberculosis

92
Unilateral chest pain accentuated by inspiration may be caused by
A a fractured rib
B perisplenitis
C myocardial infarction
D spontaneous pneumothorax
E acute mediastinitis

93
Wheeze
A is louder during inspiration than expiration
B may only follow exertion in certain patients
C may follow a bout of coughing in chronic bronchitics
D is of high pitch if a major bronchus is narrowed
E occurring only at night is diagnostic of left heart failure

94
Recognised causes of persistent nasal obstruction include
A enlarged adenoids
B nasal polypi
C mucosal oedema
D excessive secretions
E deflected nasal septum

95
Chest pain due to
A mediastinal tumour may resemble cardiac pain
B pleurisy usually worsens as an effusion develops
C spontaneous pneumothorax may be retrosternal
D a metastatic deposit in a rib is worse on respiration
E an oesophageal lesion may radiate through to the middle of the back

96
Organic laryngeal disease causes
A a 'barking' cough
B hoarseness
C haemoptysis
D stridor
E no pain

97
Tracheal stridor
A is best heard during inspiration
B is higher in pitch than laryngeal stridor
C is always accompanied by dyspnoea
D suggests an inflammatory rather than a malignant cause
E is accentuated by coughing

98
Factors of importance in the aetiology of chronic bronchitis include
A obesity
B cigarette smoking
C myelomatosis
D atmospheric pollution
E psychological maladjustment

99
Recurrent pneumonia may be aetiologically related to
A primary tuberculosis
B severe whooping cough in childhood
C bronchial carcinoma
D previous traumatic pneumothorax
E cystic fibrosis

100
The following statements about pulmonary complications of surgery are correct:
A Pulmonary abscess may develop after dental extraction due to inhalation of septic material
B Atelectasis is more likely to occur after lower than after upper abdominal operations
C Pulmonary infarction is only likely to occur after abdominal operations
D Tonsillectomy will be uncomplicated as long as it is done under general anaesthesia
E It is usual to find a persistently impaired percussion note at the lung base after thoracotomy

101
The following statements are correct:
A Bronchiectasis is a recognised sequel of post-primary but not of primary tuberculosis
B The duration of a history of recurrent pneumonia is of differential diagnostic significance
C Bronchial carcinoma is rare in non-smokers
D Pneumonia is a recognised complication of measles
E Drug allergy may be manifest as bronchial asthma

102
Recognised causes of central cyanosis include
A fibrosing alveolitis
B superior vena caval obstruction
C chronrc obstructive airways disease
D polycythaemia
E pneumonia

103
In a patient with clubbing of the fingers
A the presence of an enlarged liver gives a clue to its aetiology
B curvature of the nail in its long axis precedes shininess of the skin at the base of the nail
C pain in the forearm suggests a malabsorption syndrome
D there may be a familial trait
E the presence of clubbing of the toes makes bronchial carcinoma the most likely cause

104
Clinical findings on which a diagnosis of finger clubbing can be confidently based include
A increased curvature of the nails
B fluctuation at the nail bases
C loss of the angle between the nail and the nail base
D pitting oedema of the fingers
E swelling of the finger pulp in all dimensions

105
In a patient with respiratory disease it may be aetiologically relevant that he
A overeats
B is about to take his 'O' levels
C works on a farm
D has been exposed to asbestos
E keeps pigeons

106
Finger clubbing is a recognised feature of
A chronic bronchitis
B aortic aneurysm
C fibrosing alveolitis
D infective endocarditis
E Crohn's disease

107
The following are recognised associations:
A iridocyclitis and sarcoidosis
B choroidal tubercles and miliary tuberculosis
C phlyctenular keratoconjunctivitis and bronchiectasis
D papilloedema and arterial hypoxaemia
E conjunctival chemosis and superior vena caval obstruction

108
The following statements are correct:
A The cervical lymph nodes most commonly involved in bronchial carcinoma are those lying along the lateral border of the sternomastoid
B The cause of cervical lymph node enlargement may sometimes be determined by radiography
C Lupus vulgaris is commonly associated with pulmonary tuberculosis
D Erythema nodosum may be the initial clinical manifestation of sarcoidosis
E Lupus erythematosus may occur in association with intrathoracic sarcoidosis

109
Palpable tracheal shift to the right occurs in the presence of
A right pneumothorax
B collapse of the lung following occlusion of the right main bronchus
C right upper lobe fibrosis
D a large left pleural effusion
E right lower lobe pneumonia

110
An increased anteroposterior chest diameter may result from
A thoracic kyphosis
B chronic bronchitis with emphysema
C asthma
D thoracoplasty
E pectus excavatum

111
The following statements are correct:
A Lupus pernio is due to cutaneous involvement by carcinoma
B Subcutaneous emphysema is a recognised complication of tension pneumothorax
C The trachea moves upwards during inspiration in patients with chronic airways obstruction
D Pectus excavatum is an important cause of right heart failure
E Facial oedema is a recognised manifestation of mediastinal tumour

112
On laryngoscopy
A a clear view may be obtained of the arytenoid region as well as the vocal cords
B a laryngoscope is usually needed if a biopsy is to be taken
C a benzocaine lozenge sucked by the patient prior to examination may enable a better view to be obtained
D it is best for the patient not to protrude the tongue
E failure of a vocal cord to adduct on phonation means that it is paralysed

113
An increase in the depth of respiration is a recognised manifestation of
A ankylosing spondylitis
B diabetic ketosis
C emphysema
D cerebral haemorrhage
E uraemia

114
Respiratory movements are mainly abdominal in
A pregnancy
B normal men
C ankylosing spondylitis
D normal babies
E peritonitis

115
On palpation of the chest
A restriction of inspiratory movement is a feature of diffuse pulmonary fibrosis
B vocal fremitus is absent over a pleural effusion
C a persistent unilateral palpable rhonchus is suggestive of partial bronchial obstruction
D a palpable pleural rub is more common in acute than in chronic pleurisy
E respiratory movement in the infraclavicular regions can be gauged accurately

116
Percussion
A below the anterior end of the fourth rib may be helpful in the diagnosis of middle lobe consolidation
B over the clavicle should be over its lateral third
C produces a note over a pleural effusion which is different from that over a consolidated lobe
D should generally be from a region of normal resonance to one of impaired resonance
E of the upper border of hepatic dullness may be helpful in the diagnosis of phrenic nerve paralysis

117
On percussion of the chest
A there is resonance over a thin walled cavity
B there is resonance over the supraclavicular fossae
C dullness at the right base anteriorly corresponds to the upper level of the hepatic shadow on a PA chest radiograph
D generalised hyper-resonance is diagnostic of emphysema
E there is normally an area of impairment to the left of the lower sternum due to the heart

118
The conditions which must be satisfied before breath sounds can be described as bronchial are:
A Both the inspiratory and expiratory sounds must be blowing in character
B The expiratory sound must be as loud and long as the inspiratory sound
C The sounds must be high-pitched
D There must be no pause between the end of the inspiratory sound and the beginning of the expiratory sound
E The sounds must have a 'resonating' quality

119
On auscultation of the chest coughing will usually modify the added sounds due to
A 'dry' pleurisy
B obstruction of a large bronchus by tumour
C pneumonia
D fibrosing alveolitis
E pulmonary oedema

120
Vocal resonance is increased in
A lobar pneumonia
B localised fibrosis
C empyema
D pneumothorax
E emphysema

121
The following investigations and diseases are appropriately matched:
A tomography and chronic bronchitis
B mediastinoscopy and hilar lymphadenopathy
C fluoroscopy and diaphragmatic paralysis
D pleural biopsy and an unexplained pleural effusion
E lung biopsy and suspected fibrosing alveolitis

122
One of the most reliable methods of making a diagnosis of
A pulmonary tuberculosis is by the tuberculin test
B sarcoidosis is by the Kveim test
C pulmonary cavitation is by tomography
D bronchiectasis is by bronchography
E bronchial carcinoma is by bronchoscopy

123
The FEV$_1$/FVC ratio
A is normally about 40 per cent
B is reduced in emphysema
C is above normal in diffuse pulmonary fibrosis
D is useful in the assessment of the same aspects of respiratory disorder as the PEFR
E is the most convenient test of respiratory function for use in general practice

CHAPTER SEVEN

124
The following statements are correct:
A Waterbrash is due to regurgitation of gastric contents
B The patient's localisation of dysphagia to the lower oesophagus is a good indication of the level of the lesion
C Vomiting without preceding nausea is characteristic of migraine
D Individual bowel habit varies normally from once in 2–3 days to 2–3 times a day
E Globus hystericus is associated with upper dysphagia

125
The following may occur in the absence of any structural abnormality of the gastrointestinal tract:
A acid regurgitation
B belching
C borborygmi
D epigastric fullness after a large meal
E lower dysphagia

126
Pain associated with hiatus hernia
A is alleviated by swallowing hot fluids
B is relieved by standing
C does not occur unless peptic oesophagitis is present
D may mimic that of ischaemic heart disease
E responds poorly to alkalies

127
The pain associated with a perforated peptic ulcer may be simulated by
A acute pancreatitis
B biliary pain
C tabetic crisis
D lead 'colic'
E perisplenitis

128
Abdominal pain
A is a recognised feature of diabetic ketoacidosis
B if due to a lesion in the distal hemicolon, is localised in the left lumbar region
C associated with lead poisoning is relieved by antispasmodic drugs
D occurring after meals is a feature of chronic mid-gut ischaemia
E due to acute appendicitis may be aggravated by abduction of the right hip

129
Renal pain
A is characteristically situated in the iliac fossa
B associated with rigors suggests acute pyelonephritis
C caused by ureteric calculus is due to a rise of pressure in the renal pelvis
D is absent in polycystic disease
E may occur in association with carcinoma of the kidney if the renal capsule is stretched

130
The following statements are correct:
A Bladder dilatation with dribbling incontinence is a characteristic feature of tabes dorsalis
B The most common neurological cause of urgency of micturition is lumbar disc protrusion
C Overdistension of the urinary bladder is a recognised complication of an acute cerebrovascular accident
D Oliguria is defined as a urine output of less than 1 litre daily
E Pneumaturia is a characteristic feature of vesico-colic fistula

131
An osmotic diuresis is principally responsible for polyuria accompanying
A psychogenic polydipsia
B the use of thiazide diuretics
C chronic renal failure
D hyperparathyroidism
E diabetes mellitus

132
In an adult female a pathological process is indicated if inspection of the abdomen shows

A superficial epigastric veins draining towards the groin

B haemangiomas (Campbell de Morgan spots)

C white striae

D gastric peristalsis

E black warts

133
The following normal structures may be palpable in a healthy subject:

A liver

B right kidney

C spleen

D duodenum

E sigmoid colon

134
On palpation of the abdomen

A renal tenderness is typically most marked anteriorly

B the position of the kidneys is unaffected by breathing

C a grossly enlarged spleen is characterised by the presence of one or more notches on the anterior edge

D the fingers cannot be inserted deep to an enlarged kidney

E enlargement of the gall-bladder in the presence of jaundice is characteristic of a stone in the common bile duct

135
Percussion of the abdomen

A reveals central dullness in the presence of ascites

B is likely to lead to an overestimation of the size of the liver

C may demonstrate loss of liver dullness in the presence of a perforated peptic ulcer

D is more reliable than palpation in assessing the size of an enlarged spleen

E characteristically shows shifting dullness in the presence of a large ovarian cyst

136
The following statements are correct:

A Both indirect and direct inguinal hernias may extend into the scrotum

B A cough impulse can be felt over a saphenous varix

C A femoral hernia lies below the pubic tubercle whereas an indirect inguinal hernia lies above

D Torsion of the testis may produce signs which resemble those of a strangulated hernia

E Following reduction, pressure over the mid-inguinal point will obliterate the cough impulse in a direct inguinal hernia but not an indirect hernia

137
During examination of the male genitalia

A the presence of a hydrocele may obscure a testicular tumour

B firm, nodular enlargement of the testis is characteristic of tuberculous infection

C shortening of the spermatic cord is characteristic of torsion of the testis

D malposition of the urethral orifice may be expected in approximately five per cent of otherwise normal males

E infection with mumps virus typically causes thickening of the epididymis and cord

138
When digital examination of the rectum is performed in a male

A an abnormally small prostate is a recognised feature of Klinefelter's syndrome

B normal seminal vesicles are palpable

C piles are not palpable unless they are thrombosed

D palpation of the prostate may produce a desire to pass urine

E ballooning of the lower rectum suggests the possibility of an obstructing carcinoma in the upper rectum

139
In the investigation of disease of the liver and biliary tract
A estimation of the serum alkaline phosphatase activity is a useful test of the integrity of the liver cells
B ultrasonography can distinguish between a tumour and a liquid containing mass
C tests for hepatitis B surface antigen should be made in patients suspected of cirrhosis as well as in those with viral hepatitis
D it must be borne in mind that many gall stones are radiotranslucent
E radio-isotope scanning is incapable of detecting focal lesions less than 5cm in diameter

140
In the investigation of pancreatic disease
A a raised serum amylase is pathognomonic of acute pancreatitis
B malabsorption due to diffuse small intestinal disease may be distinguished from that due to pancreatic disease by a glucose tolerance test
C A plain abdominal X-ray in a patient with acute pancreatitis may show absence of gas in the middle of the transverse colon
D undigested meat fibres observed on microscopic examination of the faeces suggest a lack of secretion of pancreatic juice
E achlorhydria is a typical feature of the Zollinger-Ellison syndrome

141
The following statements are correct:
A Symmetrically enlarged kidneys suggest chronic parenchymal disease
B Estimation of blood creatinine gives a better indication of glomerular filtration rate than does a creatinine clearance determination
C Radio-isotope studies give no information about renal function
D The right ureteric orifice is not normally visible on cystoscopy
E A difference in size between the two kidneys may usefully be assessed by a plain X-ray film of the abdomen

142
In a patient who is suspected to be suffering from an 'acute abdomen'
A severe pain should be alleviated by analgesics before physical examination is commenced
B a perforated duodenal ulcer is characterised by restlessness
C basal pneumonia may mimic an acute abdominal emergency
D acute peritonitis is characterised by abnormally loud bowel sounds
E visible peristalsis is a feature of intestinal obstruction

CHAPTER EIGHT

143
The following are 'hard' (reliable) signs of organic disease in the nervous system:
A the patient's failure to respond to pinching of the calf muscles
B an extensor plantar response
C extensive sensory loss unaccompanied by symptoms
D Chvostek's sign
E an absent 'gag' reflex

144
Observation of the patient's face during the taking of the history may give information which leads to the diagnosis of
A epilepsy
B Parkinsonism
C myasthenia gravis
D chorea
E myopathy

145
The following are correct definitions:
A Dysphasia: inability to enunciate words clearly
B Dysphonia: inability to speak other than in a whisper
C Dyslexia: impaired ability to read
D Dysarthria: inability to write
E Dysgraphia: inability to interpret visual information

146
Dysphonia may be the consequence of
A myasthenia gravis
B supranuclear bulbar palsy
C Parkinsonism
D cerebellar disease
E a lesion of the speech area in the dominant hemisphere

147
The speech area in the brain
A is on the right side in the great majority of left-handed subjects
B is the site of damage in dysarthric patients
C is usually on the side opposite to that of the dominant eye
D includes the superior temporal gyrus
E exhibits characteristic pathological changes in patients who stammer

148
Characteristic findings in myasthenia gravis include
A ptosis
B absent pupillary reflexes
C dysphasia
D improvement after injection of edrophonium
E muscular wasting

149
The following are recognised causes of dysarthria:
A myopathy
B myasthenia gravis
C interruption of both recurrent laryngeal nerves
D supranuclear bulbar palsy
E cerebellar disease

150
Characteristic findings in Parkinsonism include
A failure to swing the arm while walking
B a festinant gait
C an ataxic gait with constant veering towards one side
D nystagmus
E cogwheel rigidity

151
Anosmia
A is more commonly due to neurological causes than to nasal disease
B may be described by the patient as a loss of taste
C may be a consequence of head injury
D when suspected, should be confirmed by testing with ammonia or vinegar
E may be caused by intracranial tumours

152
A right homonymous hemianopia could be satisfactorily explained by
A damage to the right optic nerve
B pressure on the optic chiasma
C a lesion of the left optic tract
D a lesion of the right occipital cortex
E a lesion involving the left lateral geniculate body

153
Total paralysis of the third cranial nerve causes, on the same side,
A dilatation of the pupil
B ptosis
C paralysis of lateral gaze
D absence of facial sweating
E absence of the accommodation reflex

154
The superior oblique muscle
A is supplied by the fourth cranial nerve
B causes the eye to look down during lateral gaze
C combines with the inferior rectus to produce downward gaze without deflection
D causes the eye to look up during medial gaze
E commonly becomes paralysed as a result of increased intracranial pressure

155
Conjugate deviation of the eyes requires the intact functioning of
A the medial longitudinal bundle
B fibres connecting the frontal area to the pontine region
C the occipital cortex
D the superior oblique muscle of the abducting eye
E the inferior rectus muscle of the adducting eye

156
The following structures pass through the cavernous sinus:
A the internal carotid artery
B the oculomotor nerve
C the trochlear nerve
D the abducent nerve
E the mandibular division of the trigeminal nerve

157
Paralysis of the lateral rectus muscle of the eye could be a consequence of
A a posterior fossa tumour
B Wernicke's encephalopathy
C an intracranial aneurysm in the cavernous sinus
D damage to the cervical sympathetic outflow
E a lesion in the pons

158
The cervical sympathetic outflow
A supplies the sphincter pupillae
B supplies the orbital muscle which tends to hold the eye forward in the orbit
C supplies the levator palpebrae superioris
D supplies the sweat-glands of the skin of the face
E leaves the spinal cord via the first two or three thoracic roots

159
In testing a patient's eye movements you observe that when he looks to the right there is satisfactory abduction of the right eye, but poor adduction of the left eye. The explanation could be
A a weakness of the left superior rectus muscle
B a weakness of the left medial rectus muscle
C a lesion of the medial longitudinal bundle
D a lesion of the left sixth cranial nerve
E a lesion of the cerebellum

160
Drooping of an upper eyelid may be due to a lesion of the
A levator palpebrae muscle
B third cranial nerve
C parabducens nucleus
D cervical sympathetic outflow
E seventh cranial nerve

161
In testing a patient's eye movements you find that he experiences diplopia with wide separation between the images on looking upwards and to the right. Covering and uncovering the right and left eye separately establishes that the image displaced in the direction of gaze is that seen by the right eye. These findings could indicate a weakness of the

A right lateral rectus
B left superior rectus
C right superior rectus
D right inferior oblique
E right superior oblique

162
In testing a patient's pupillary response you observe the following:

Light shone into	Response of	
	Right pupil	Left pupil
Right eye	None	None
Left eye	Constriction	Constriction

The following explanations are compatible with these findings:
A paralysis of right third cranial nerve
B adhesions from old iritis in the right eye
C damage to the right optic nerve
D tonic pupillary reaction (Holmes-Adie syndrome)
E Argyll-Robertson pupil on the right

163
The following are recognised findings in disorders of the cerebellum:
A scanning dysarthria
B increased muscular tone in the limbs
C intention tremor
D pendular nystagmus
E past-pointing

164
While examining a patient's eye movements you observe nystagmus when he looks to his left, but not in any other direction of gaze. The left eye only is affected and the fast component is to the left. Adduction of the right eye on looking to the left is incomplete. The cause may be
A defective macular vision in the left eye
B vestibular neuronitis on the left side
C a lesion of the left cerebellar hemisphere
D a lesion of the medial longitudinal bundle
E damage to the semicircular canals on the left side

165
Impaired facial sensation is a recognised consequence of
A herpes zoster
B trigeminal neuralgia
C an acoustic neuroma
D a lesion of the internal capsule
E an intracranial aneurysm

166
Recognised features of an upper motor neurone facial weakness include
A drooping of the angle of the mouth
B inability to wrinkle the forehead
C preservation of emotional smiling
D weakness of the masseter muscle
E ptosis

167
The descending (spinal) tract of the fifth cranial nerve
A descends as far as the fifth cervical segment of the cord
B conveys sensory impulses from pain and temperature receptors
C conveys motor impulses to the pterygoid muscles
D gives rise to fibres which decussate and pass to the thalamus
E does not conform in the grouping of its fibres to the three main divisions of the nerve

168
The integrity of tracts in the spinal cord may be tested effectively by the procedures named:
A lateral spino-thalamic tract: touching the skin with a point of cotton wool which is not moved across the skin
B posterior columns: testing joint position sense at the great toe
C pyramidal tract: testing abdominal reflexes
D extrapyramidal system: carrying out the heel-knee test
E spinal tract of the fifth cranial nerve: testing pain sensation over the forehead

169
Transection of the seventh cranial nerve as it leaves the stylomastoid foramen will cause, on the same side,
A inability to wrinkle the forehead
B loss of taste over the anterior two-thirds of the tongue
C development of a 'snout reflex'
D upward deviation of the eye on attempting to close the eyelids
E hyperacusis

170
Examination of a 60-year old patient complaining of deafness of the right ear shows that Weber's test is referred to the left (heard most loudly in the left ear) and Rinne's test on the right gives a normal response (air conduction better than bone conduction). The reason for the deafness might be
A old age
B wax in the auditory meatus
C an acoustic neuroma
D chronic otitis media
E Ménière's syndrome

171
Recognised features of pseudo-bulbar palsy include
A dysarthria
B exaggerated jaw-jerk
C bilateral wasting of the tongue with fasciculation
D dysphagia
E emotional lability

172
Fasciculation of muscle
A represents the spontaneous contractions of single muscle fibres
B always implies the presence of serious disease
C suggests lower motor neurone rather than upper motor neurone involvement
D may occur in the absence of wasting of the muscle
E does not occur in the tongue

173
The following signs constitute reliable evidence of upper motor neurone damage:
A extensor plantar responses
B absent abdominal reflexes
C positive Rossolimo's sign
D generalised increase in tendon reflexes
E sustained ankle clonus

174
The following are recognised signs of disease of the extrapyramidal system:
A 'lead-pipe' rigidity
B intention tremor
C delay in initiation of movements
D delayed relaxation of tendon reflexes
E athetosis

175
Dyspraxia
A is correctly defined as inability to carry out simple movements because of muscular inco-ordination
B may be confused clinically with hysteria
C is very often associated with dysphasia
D should be sought by means of the finger-nose test
E could be explained as a consequence of a lesion in one or other parietal lobe

176
The lateral spino-thalamic tract of the spinal cord
A transmits temperature sensation from the opposite side of the body
B transmits pain sensation from the same side of the body
C is not involved in the transmission of the sensation of light touch
D is laminated so that fibres from the lowest spinal segments lie outermost
E runs directly to the thalamus without relay in the cord

177

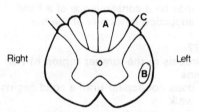

Right   Left

Sensations are conveyed in the spinal cord as indicated in the diagram:
A vibration sense from the left: A
B position sense from the left: B
C temperature sensation from the right: B
D vibration sense from the left: C
E touch from the right: A

178
The following are correct descriptions:
A Kernig's sign: inability to stand upright with the heels together and the eyes closed
B Barber's chair sign: tingling down the back and limbs when the head is bent forward
C Trousseau's sign: contraction of facial muscles following a tap over the facial nerve in front of the ear
D Rossolimo's sign: plantar flexion of the great toe when the remaining toes are flicked into extension by the examiner
E Hoffman's sign: flexion of finger joints when the supinator jerk is elicited

179
Loss of tendon reflexes
A occurs early in the course of myopathies
B occurs late in peripheral neuropathy
C does not usually occur in myasthenia
D in the biceps, may be accompanied by inversion
E is not necessarily pathological

180
An absent plantar response may be due to
A cold feet
B sensory impairment in the S1 distribution
C use of too sharp a point in eliciting the response
D paralysis of flexor or extensor hallucis longus
E spinal shock

181
Recognised manifestations of hypocalcaemia include
A main d'accoucheur
B a positive Trousseau's sign
C a positive cremasteric reflex
D a positive Chvosteko's sign
E absent abdominal reflexes

182
The following c.s.f. results are acceptable as normal findings on lumbar puncture:
A Appearance : clear and faintly yellow coloured
B Cells: 20 lymphocytes per cubic millimetre
C Protein: 0.2g/l
D Glucose: 3.0mmol/l
E IgG: 50% of total protein

183
Electroencephalography
A is more precise in its definition of hemisphere than of posterior fossa lesions
B shows more marked changes with acute than with chronic lesions
C is the most effective way of deciding whether or not a patient is epileptic
D is more effective in detecting gliomas than meningiomas
E is best avoided until after any necessary intracranial contrast radiography has been completed

184
Computerised Assisted Tomography (CAT scan)
A takes about four hours to perform
B involves the injection of radioactive tracers
C exposes the patient to less radiation than that of an ordinary skull X-ray
D is useful in the diagnosis of cerebral abscess
E commonly gives rise to severe headache for some days afterwards

185
A diagnosis of brain death is supported by
A pin-point pupils
B absent corneal reflexes
C sluggish eye movements after the injection of ice-cold water into the external auditory meati
D the absence of spontaneous respiration even when PCO_2 is greater than 6.6 kPa (50 mmHg)
E the absence of electrical activity of cerebral origin on the e.e.g.

CHAPTER NINE

186
Scoliosis
A is normal in children who have just begun to walk
B if postural is corrected on flexion of the spine
C if due to a painful condition is associated with limited flexion of the spine
D if due to a painless structural lesion persists on flexion
E may be a consequence of a fixed adduction deformity of the hip

187
Lordosis in the lumbar region of the spine
A does not appear until a child begins to walk
B diminishes during pregnancy
C is more marked in a young adult than in a toddler
D is known as a gibbus when it is unduly marked
E disappears if the lumbar discs degenerate

188
The term
A genu valgum is applied to any condition in which the tibiae are not parallel
B varus is applied to a deviation at a joint towards the midline
C cubitus valgus is used to describe the normal female elbow
D genu varum is applied to a bow-leg deformity
E talipes implies a deformity involving the ankle and foot

189
The gait of a patient
A with a painful knee is disturbed in contour rather than in rhythm
B with ankylosis of the hip without deformity may be normal
C with a stiff knee is characterised by descent of stairs with the sound leg leading
D with myopathy of the gluteal muscles is described as 'waddling'
E with a below-knee prosthesis is described as 'peg leg'

190
The following statements about joint movement are correct:
A Raising the arm vertically is mostly due to movement of the scapula
B Hand movements are normal if the patient can fully flex the fingers to form a closed fist
C Weakness of the serratus anterior muscle may result in 'winging' of the scapula
D If rotation of the hip is unimpaired, it is unlikely that other significant limitation is present
E Records of joint movement which are not expressed quantitatively are useless

191
In the Neutral Zero method for recording joint movements the neutral position of the
A hands is with the palms facing forwards
B feet is at right angles to the leg
C elbow is maximal extension
D hip is the natural position of the erect stance
E fingers is flexion into a fist

192
The following statements are correct:
A A strained ligament is painful when actively stretched towards the opposite side of the joint
B A strained ligament leads to tenderness over the entire affected joint
C If dorsiflexion of the ankle is possible only when the knee is flexed, contracture of the gastrocnemius is a probable diagnosis
D Joint effusions are exceptional following tearing of a semilunar cartilage
E Differentiation of pain from torn muscles as opposed to a strained ligament can be made if isometric contraction is painful

193
Pain
A occurring immediately after an acute ligamentous strain is only felt on movement
B in the back due to chronic ligamentous strain is worst in the early morning
C on movement may be absent if a fracture is impacted
D caused by acute joint suppuration may wake the patient suddenly at night
E characteristically worsens during the day in patients with rheumatoid disease

194
The following statements are correct:
A A malingerer usually produces a bizarre, apparently painless, gait
B Pain is an invariable feature of malignant tumours of bone
C An osteoid osteoma is typically painless
D Acute prolapse of an intervertebral disc usually occurs in a patient who has not previously had back pain
E Intermittent claudication and pain due to osteoarthrosis are both quickly relieved by rest

195
The following muscles are supplied by the nerves named:
A short flexor of the thumb—radial nerve
B opponens pollicis—median nerve
C the lumbrical to the ring finger—median nerve
D finger extensors—radial nerve
E adductor pollicis—ulnar nerve

196
The hand
A is capable of gripping firmly even without the help of the intrinsic muscles
B has an almost constant distribution of its nerve supply
C is rarely affected by rheumatoid disease
D becomes clawed if the ulnar nerve is damaged
E is incapable of sorting change in the pocket if the median nerve is paralysed

197
The following associations are correct:
A tenderness in the 'anatomical snuff-box' and scaphoid fracture
B limitation of flexion and 'trigger-finger'
C humeral neck fracture and wrist-drop
D supracondylar fracture of the humerus and ischaemic changes in the flexor muscles of the forearm
E rupture of the extensor pollicis longus tendon and rheumatoid arthritis

198
During examination of the elbow
A the collateral ligaments can be tested only when the elbow is fully flexed
B in 'tennis elbow' tenderness is localised in the region of the medial epicondyle
C an effusion is most easily felt over the head of the radius on the postero-lateral aspect of the joint
D the ulnar nerve should also be examined
E a flexion deformity can be differentiated easily from a valgus deformity

199
Pain in the shoulder
A is most commonly due to a lesion in the supraspinatus tendon
B may be caused by diaphragmatic pleurisy even though the shoulder is stiff on examination
C due to an apical bronchial carcinoma radiates down the outer arm to the insertion of the deltoid muscle
D resulting from myocardial ischaemia is referred to the tip of the shoulder
E may be severe enough to demand immediate operation in some rotator cuff lesions

200
A lesion of the rotator cuff may be manifested by
A pain in the shoulder during resisted flexion of the elbow
B pain in the shoulder during abduction
C inability to hold the arm abducted to 90°
D inability to shrug the shoulder
E recurrent dislocation of the shoulder

201
The cervical spine is
A the most mobile section of the vertebral column
B a common site of crush fracture of a vertebra
C only rarely the site of a congenital deformity
D an unusual site for disc protrusion
E particularly liable to dislocation in forced flexion injury of the neck

202
The thoracic spine is
A normally kyphotic
B only rarely affected by tuberculosis
C the commonest site of symptomatic intervertebral disc lesions
D more mobile in rotation than in flexion and extension
E sometimes so severely scoliotic that cardiac and respiratory function is impaired

203
The following statements are correct:
A The lumbosacral region is a common site for painless congenital anomalies
B The spinal cord ends at the level of L4
C A vestigial rib may be mistaken radiologically for a fractured lumbar transverse process
D Pus from osteomyelitis of a lumbar vertebra tends to surface between the spinous processes and the erector spinae muscle
E Passive flexion of the hip aggravates the pain of psoas abscess

204
The following are aetiologically related:
A gluteal pain on exercise and occlusive arterial disease
B pain only at the end of the day and osteoarthrosis
C low back pain and ankylosing spondylitis
D pain over the sacrum and malignant uterine tumour
E pain on pressure between the lumbar laminae and prolapsed disc

205
In a patient with a prolapsed intervertebral disc
A impaired straight leg raising suggests an L2/3 disc protrusion
B at the limit of straight leg raising further root tension may be achieved by forced dorsiflexion of the ankle
C disc protrusion at the L2/3 level may prevent him lying prone
D the side to which a patient leans indicates the relation of the disc protrusion to the nerve root
E pain due to involvement of the roots of the femoral nerve is exacerbated by extending the hip with the knee flexed

206
A fixed hip deformity
A in flexion is associated with a decreased lumbar lordosis
B in flexion is compensated by raising the heel of the affected leg
C in abduction is compensated by raising the foot on the normal side
D in adduction is compensated by bending the knee to the affected side
E in a combination of adduction and flexion is commoner than any single deformity

207
Dislocation of the hip
A is commoner as a congenital abnormality than dislocation of the shoulder
B in infants is most likely to occur when the joint is extended and adducted
C is most likely to occur in adults when the joint is flexed
D in a posterior direction causes the leg to be externally rotated and abducted
E in an anterior direction causes the leg to be internally rotated and adducted

208
Recognised features of unilateral congenital dislocation of the hip include
A shortening of the limb
B relative lack of spontaneous movement on the affected side
C asymmetry of the thigh and buttock folds
D limitation of hip abduction
E internal rotation of the limb

209
In the knee joint
A the normal range of movement is 0–150°
B the semilunar cartilages are prone to damage because they are immobile
C stability depends more on muscles and ligaments than on the shape of the bones
D the cruciate ligaments tighten in full flexion
E a violent blow on one side in extension is liable to cause rupture of the opposite collateral ligament

210
On examination of the knee joint
A patellar tap is the most sensitive sign of a small effusion
B the collateral ligaments should be tested in extension
C the integrity of the cruciate ligaments is tested by assessing the antero-posterior 'glide' of the tibia with the knee at right angles
D the presence of crepitus is diagnostic of intra-articular loose bodies
E visible bruising confined to one side suggests a cartilage injury

211
The following statements about the leg and foot are correct:
A With the patient kneeling, gentle squeezing of the calf distal to its maximal circumference can differentiate between rupture of the tendo Archillis and avulsion of the medial head of gastrocnemius
B Talipes equinovarus means that the ankle and foot are plantar flexed and the foot adducted and inverted
C Pes planus is usually accompanied by varus deformity at the ankle
D When the lateral ligament of the ankle is torn the abnormal movement of the talus in the ankle mortice can only be detected by radiography
E Ischaemia can be excluded as a cause of pain in the foot if the pain is not made worse by exercise

212
Rupture of the tendo Achillis
A causes total loss of active plantar flexion of the foot
B causes excessive passive dorsiflexion of the foot
C has no effect on active dorsiflexion of the foot
D is typically accompanied by a palpable gap in the tendon
E must be confirmed by radiological investigation

213
Regarding investigation of the locomotor system, the following statements are correct:
A If the fragments of a simple bone fracture are in good position on the antero-posterior film, there is no need to subject the patient to the discomfort of a lateral radiograph
B A suspected fractured scaphoid should be treated in plaster even in the presence of negative radiographs
C The epiphysis may be confused with a fracture on X-ray of the elbow in children
D An arthrogram may be helpful in diagnosing injuries to semilunar cartilages
E Bone scanning can detect neoplastic lesions which are not visible radiologically

214
A patient should be suspected of malingering if he
A complains of pain consistently relieved by rest
B describes pain of an absolutely symmetrical distribution
C can make a fist even though he complains of a 'dropped wrist'
D is very quick to take the weight off the limb in which he complains of pain
E tends to show a pattern of anaesthesia the distribution of which is similar to that of polyneuritis

CHAPTER TEN

215
Problems arising in obtaining the history of a young child are that the parents may
A interpret rather than describe clinical events
B explain the present illness in terms of a diagnosis assigned to a past one
C be unaware that the child's description of his own symptoms is inaccurate
D fail to realise that their behaviour may be contributing to the illness of an emotionally disturbed child
E overestimate the child's calorie intake, especially that taken in liquid form

216
The presence of the following manifestations may shed light on the origin of abdominal pain in a child:
A melaena
B sore throat
C cough
D purpura
E constipation

217
In taking a paediatric history, you should be more than usually alert to the possibility of important organic disease if the mother says that she has noticed
A pallor during sleep
B convulsions
C blueness of the lips
D difficulty in swallowing
E increased volume of urine

218
In examining a child
A the best time to take the blood pressure is at the beginning of the examination
B if the child behaves badly the doctor should ask the mother to control him
C it is best not to depart from a clear-cut routine of examination
D gentle stroking of the skin with one finger may quieten the child
E the child should always be placed on an examination couch

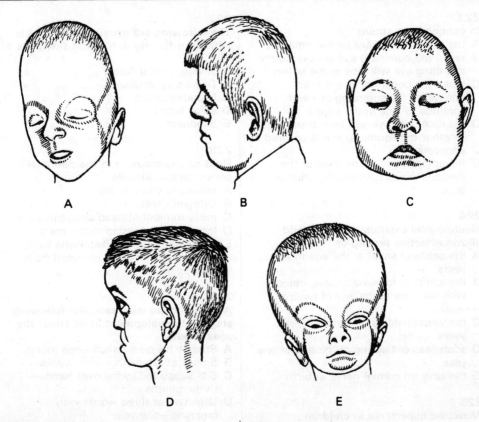

A   B   C

D   E

219
Inspection of a child's face and head may give important information in connection with
A renal agenesis
B cretinism
C liver disease
D myasthenia gravis
E spina bifida

220
The appearances of a child's head as shown in the diagrams above should raise suspicions that the following may be present:
Diagram A craniostenosis
Diagram B Turner's syndrome
Diagram C mental retardation
Diagram D rickets
Diagram E spina bifida.

221
In a baby's head
A the posterior fontanelle is normally closed at one month
B the anterior fontanelle should still be open at one year
C an increase in tension in the anterior fontanelle is normal unless the head is enlarged
D it is normally possible to indent the skull bones with light finger pressure
E the sagittal suture is identifiable at birth

222
If a child is crying it is not worthwhile trying to
A auscultate the breath sounds
B auscultate the heart sounds
C palpate the abdomen
D count the respiratory rate
E detect a facial paralysis

223
In concomitant squint
A the squint is present all the time
B when the dominant eye is covered the squinting eye will look at the object
C when the dominant eye is then uncovered the squinting eye will continue to look at the object
D the dominant eye will look at the object whether the squinting eye is covered or uncovered
E the angle between the axes of the eyeballs varies with the direction of gaze

224
Neurological examination in a child allows effective testing of
A the sense of smell at the age of two years
B the ability to follow a moving object with the eyes at the age of twelve weeks
C the visual fields at the age of three years
D acuteness of hearing at the age of one year
E the seventh cranial nerve at birth

225
Muscular hypertonia in children
A is usually of the 'clasp knife' variety
B is nearly always generalised
C is often particularly marked in the adductors of the thigh
D seldom affects the plantar flexor muscles of the foot severely
E is accompanied by excessive firmness of the muscles

226
The following reflexes are normally seen in babies at the ages given:
A Moro reflex at six months
B grasp reflex at one month
C rooting reflex at two weeks
D tonic neck reflex at five months
E light reflex at three days

227
The following are usually recognisable without difficulty in the first few days of life:
A severe mental defect
B Down's syndrome
C hypothyroidism
D spina bifida
E blindness

228
Routine examination in the neonatal period should include
A testing of visual fields
B Ortolani's test
C measurement of head circumference
D localisation of testes in the male
E screening for phenylketonuria by examination of blood obtained from heel pricks

229
A normal child will reach the following stages of development at or about the ages given:
A Studies his own hands—one month
B Smiles at his mother—six weeks
C Sits supported by his own hands— three months
D Uses two or three words with meaning—one year
E Can count up to ten—three years

CHAPTER ELEVEN

230
When using an ophthalmoscope
A the environment should be darkened whenever possible
B the use of mydriatics should be followed by eserine drops to reduce the risk of glaucoma
C the patient should be asked not to blink
D inspection of the macula may be facilitated by narrowing the beam of light
E the head of the instrument should not be closer than 6 inches from the patient's pupil

231
Ophthalmoscopic findings which are of no clinical significance include
A an indistinct nasal disc margin
B a dull red patch, darker than the surrounding retina, at the macula
C broad white brush-like streaks radiating from the edge of the disc, obscuring blood vessels
D streaks of dense pigment between the main choroidal vessels
E engorgement and lack of pulsation in retinal veins

232
A retinal haemorrhage
A in the nerve fibre layer occurs in arterial hypertension
B in the deeper layers of the retina remains unchanged for many months
C in the choroid may be confused with a melanotic tumour
D in the subhyaloid space may rupture into the vitreous and obscure the fundus completely
E can result from severe anaemia

233
The following statements about ophthalmoscopy are correct:
A The iris can be examined using a 'plus' lens with a focal length of 5 cm
B If the examiner is myopic he should use a biconcave lens in his ophthalmoscope
C If the patient is myopic the disc and vessels appear very small
D A doctor should never wear spectacles when using an ophthalmoscope
E There is no method of correcting for gross astigmatism in the patient by altering the lens of the ophthalmoscope

234
Soft retinal exudates
A lie deeply within the retina
B are due to arteriolar occlusions
C disappear in a few weeks
D are a recognised sequel of choroiditis
E are of serious prognostic significance in hypertension

CHAPTER TWELVE

235
Normal urinary findings include
A a 24 hour volume of 4000 ml
B cloudiness due to phosphates
C an ammoniacal smell on standing
D a pH more acid than 6.0
E a specific gravity of 1020 in a random specimen

236
The colour of urine may be
A smoky-brown in the presence of haematuria
B reddish-orange in a patient taking phenolphthalein
C red on standing in porphyria
D dark green after eating asparagus
E dark grey as a result of therapy with methyl-dopa

237
Proteinuria
A almost always indicates the presence of disease of the kidneys
B cannot be detected with certainty by the salicylsulphonic acid test in a patient taking sulphonamides
C is best tested for by Albustix in patients on large doses of phenothiazine drugs
D due to multiple myeloma does not give a positive Albustix test
E gives an orange colour with Albustix

238
In testing for glycosuria
A Clinistix is more sensitive than Clinitest
B Clinistix may be positive in late pregnancy due to lactosuria
C ascorbic acid given therapeutically may interfere with test results
D Clinitest has the advantage over Clinistix of being quantitative
E a false positive Clinitest may occur in a deeply jaundiced patient

239
In testing the urine for ketones
A an infected urine must be tested without delay, if a false negative result is to be avoided
B the ferric chloride is the most reliable test for following the progress of a patient in diabetic ketosis
C disappearance on boiling of the reddish-brown colour of a 'positive' ferric chloride test indicates that salicylates have interfered with the test
D the urine should be heated before using Acetest tablets
E Ketostix is satisfactory as a semi-quantitative test

240
Ehrlich's aldehyde reagent is involved in the detection in the urine of
A phenylpyruvic acid
B salicylates
C porphobilinogen
D haemoglobin
E urobilinogen

241
On microscopic examination of the urine
A ova of *Schistosoma haematobium* may be identified with certainty
B red cells become shrunken and crenated in dilute urine
C pus cells are more easily recognised if a 10% solution of acetic acid is run under the cover slip
D red blood cell casts always reflect glomerular disease
E the only crystals of significant diagnostic value are those of cystine

242
Blood for haematological studies
A can be conveniently obtained by puncture of the heel in babies
B if taken by pipette is dangerous if it enters the mouth
C should be collected by venepuncture only if more than 5 ml is required
D collected by venepuncture should be mixed with potassium EDTA anticoagulant immediately
E must be examined within one hour for a platelet count

243
The erythrocyte sedimentation rate
A rises with increasing age
B is always raised in patients with myeloma
C needs to be corrected if iron-deficiency anaemia is present
D is very low in polycythaemia
E is usually raised in cardiac failure

244
In preparing a blood film
A a chemically clean slide must be used
B the slide should be polished with a grease-free cloth
C a spreading slide should be placed at right angles to the slide bearing the patient's blood
D film thickness can be varied by varying the size of the drop of blood
E it is important to let the film dry slowly

245
Macrocytosis
A is usually accompanied by poikilocytosis in folate deficiency
B is a feature of excessive alcohol intake
C is the sequel of megaloblastic blood formation in the marrow only if there is co-existing deficiency of iron
D is a recognised consequence of hypothyroidism
E is a characteristic feature of thalassaemia

246
The following statements on the morphology of blood cells are correct:
A The nucleus of the eosinophil often resembles a pair of spectacles
B The diameter of the lymphocyte is about half that of a red cell
C The monocyte is the largest white cell
D Platelets are about the same size as red cells
E The presence of primitive white cells in the peripheral blood does not necessarily imply that the patient has leukaemia

247
In the investigation of haemorrhagic disease
A the whole blood clotting time is only prolonged when the coagulation factors are seriously deficient or inhibitors are present
B a normal bleeding time does not exclude a capillary defect
C the Fibrindex test is of limited value because it takes so long to do
D the presence of red cells resembling holly leaves is suggestive of intravascular coagulation and fibrinolysis
E the bleeding time is normal in thrombocytopenia

248
The following statements about SI units are correct:
A The litre is used as the unit of volume in laboratory work
B Equivalent concentrations (mEq/l) remain part of the SI system
C Mass concentrations (e.g. g/l) are used for all protein measurements except haemoglobin
D SI units are not employed for enzymes
E 1 fl oz is equivalent to approximately 50 ml

249
Problem-orientated medical records
A have been developed for over ten years
B include a 'profile' of how a patient spends an average day
C only include problems in which a diagnosis has been reached
D take less time to complete than traditional records
E stress the education of the patient in the management of his disease

250
Medical audit
A is aimed at higher professional
   standards
B can only be effective if it carries a
   punitive threat
C has shown that it is only necessary to
   take one reading of blood pressure
   before starting treatment for
   hypertension
D has revealed that the number of
   operations performed is more closely
   related to the number of surgeons than
   to the number of patients
E is now being used to study the cost-
   effectiveness of treatment

Section 2
MCQ on Davidson's *Principles and Practice of Medicine*

CHAPTER ONE

251
The following statements about genetic diseases are correct:
A Over a third of childhood deaths in developed countries can be attributed to genetically determined causes
B All diseases which are entirely genetic in origin show microscopically identifiable chromosomal abnormalities
C Over a thousand unifactorial genetic diseases are recognised
D Most infections are entirely environmental in aetiology
E In multifactorial disorders it is probable that many genes are involved and the risks to relatives are high

252
Deoxyribonucleic acid
A is composed of two identical polynucleotide chains
B contains the same nitrogenous bases as ribonucleic acid
C is found mainly in the chromosomes
D is coated with histone and non-histone proteins in higher organisms
E contains genetic information which is transferred to the ribosomes via transfer-RNA

253
In man
A somatic cell nuclei contain 22 pairs of homologous autosomes
B the nucleus of a sperm contains both X and Y chromosomes
C the nuclei of gametes are said to be haploid with respect to their chromosome complement
D the individual autosomes differ from each other only in their specific staining patterns
E X chromosomes are much larger than Y chromosomes

254
During mitosis
A the centromere of each chromosome divides into two
B there is an exchange of genetic material between the two chromatids of each chromosome
C 46 separate chromatids are in motion during anaphase
D the nuclear membrane disappears as the spindle appears
E the genetic material of the parent cell is exactly reproduced in both daughter cells

255
The following statements are correct:
A Meiosis results in the production of four cells each with 23 chromosomes
B Cell division can be stimulated in vitro by colchicine
C During the first meiotic division chromosomes migrate in the same way as do chromatids during mitosis
D The addition of hypotonic saline to a dividing cell arrested in metaphase causes the chromosomes to arrange themselves as a karyotype
E Mitotic studies are usually performed on cells from bone marrow

256
The cell nuclei of
A a normal male have the same number of Barr bodies as the nuclei of a patient with Turner's syndrome
B a patient with Klinefelter's syndrome contain one or more Barr bodies and an F body
C a girl with Down's syndrome have the karyotype 46, XX, +21
D polymorphonuclear leucocytes of a few females (about 3 per cent) have a small accessory lobule resembling a drumstick
E normal females contain only one active X chromosome

257

Non-disjunction of chromosomes 21 during meiosis

A results in the production of a gamete with three chromosomes 21

B occurs more often in the ova of older women

C is the cause of the great majority of cases of Down's syndrome

D is a cause of aneuploidy

E may sometimes be under genetic control

258

Characteristic features of Klinefelter's syndrome include

A gynaecomastia

B coarctation of the aorta

C sterility

D short stature

E criminal tendencies

259

Characteristic features of Turner's syndrome include

A severe mental retardation

B cubitus valgus

C webbing of the neck

D an increased tendency to develop acute leukaemia

E primary amenorrhoea

260

In a family affected by a disease transmitted by autosomal dominant inheritance

A affected individuals are usually heterozygotes

B half of the children of an affected parent are likely to be affected

C the sexes are invariably affected equally

D the disease may appear when no members of previous generations have been affected

E non-penetrance of the gene could explain freedom of a whole generation from the disease

261

If two persons heterozygous for a disease transmitted by autosomal recessive inheritance marry

A there is a 1 in 4 chance of each of their children being affected

B a few of their grandchildren will almost certainly be affected

C the chance that both of their only two children will be unaffected is slightly better than evens

D there is a 1 in 100 chance (in Britain) that they are first cousins

E all their healthy children will be heterozygous for the disease

262

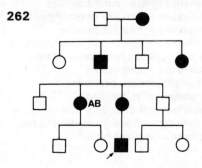

In the pedigree illustrated above

A there is unequivocal evidence that the disease is transmitted by a dominant gene

B the pattern is compatible with inheritance of an autosomal gene

C the pattern is characteristic of X-linked inheritance

D any other children subject AB has are most unlikely to be affected

E all the proband's children will be affected

263

The following statements about a male haemophiliac (married to a normal female) are correct:

A All his sisters will be carriers

B Half his daughters will be carriers

C His maternal grandfather may have suffered from the disease

D None of his sons will be affected

E One of his daughters could have haemophilia if she also has Turner's syndrome

264
The following diseases are transmitted as autosomal dominant traits:
A phenylketonuria
B polyposis of the colon
C achondroplasia
D Marfan's syndrome
E cystic fibrosis of the pancreas

265
The following diseases are transmitted as X-linked recessive traits:
A haemochromatosis
B Christmas disease
C pseudo-hypertrophic muscular dystrophy (Duchenne)
D hereditary spherocytosis
E nephrogenic diabetes insipidus

266
The risk of a child being born with congenital pyloric stenosis is greater if
A the child is a boy than if it is a girl
B the child's father had the disease than if its mother did
C two rather than one of the child's siblings had the disease
D the mother is aged 40 than if she is aged 20
E a brother was severely rather than mildly affected by the disease

267
The heritability of the first of the following pairs of diseases is greater than that of the second:
A asthma—coronary artery disease
B late onset diabetes—early onset diabetes
C congenital heart disease—schizophrenia
D congenital pyloric stenosis—peptic ulcer
E cleft lip and palate—congenital dislocation of the hip

268
When advising the parents of a child born with a congenital disorder about the risk of recurrence in subsequent children
A it may be possible, by appropriate tests, to decide that the mother is the carrier of an X-linked recessive gene
B the risk cannot be quoted precisely even for a unifactorial disorder
C the possibility that the disorder was due to intrauterine infection must be considered
D it is important to explain the exact nature of the disorder
E the parents' decision may be influenced by the efficacy of treatment for the disorder

269
Amniocentesis can be used to make an ante-natal diagnosis of
A Huntington's chorea
B Down's syndrome
C the sex of the fetus
D anencephaly
E pseudo-hypertrophic muscular dystrophy (Duchenne)

CHAPTER TWO

270
The HLA antigens
A are situated on chromosome 6
B give rise to the immune response which causes rejection of a skin graft
C are present on leucocytes
D include the genes responsible for ankylosing spondylitis
E are subdivided into four series

271
Tom and Jerry are brothers; Jemima is Jerry's wife. Skin is grafted from Jerry to Tom and Jemima
A The graft will probably survive longer in Tom than in Jemima
B A subsequent skin graft from Tom to Jerry will be rejected in 3–4 days
C A subsequent skin graft from Jemima to Tom should still be healthy after 10 days
D The graft to Jemima is known as an allograft
E A subsequent skin graft from Jerry to Jemima will become infiltrated with mononuclear cells within 3 days

272
In response to the presence of an antigen
A immunocompetent lymphocytes become transformed into lymphoblasts
B the rate of production of small lymphocytes in the thymus is increased
C the thymus begins to produce K cells
D B lymphocytes are transformed into plasma cells
E T lymphocytes react with the antigen even in the absence of free antibody

273
T lymphocytes
A circulate in the blood in smaller numbers than B lymphocytes
B are responsible for cell-mediated immunity
C are smaller than B lymphocytes
D can become transformed into K cells
E live longer than B lymphocytes

274
In the presence of a specific antigen, T lymphocytes
A release a factor which directly stimulates B lymphocytes to synthesise antibody
B prevent the antigen from coming into contact with B lymphocytes
C undergo mitosis
D release a factor which can cause other lymphocytes, not in contact with the antigen, to undergo mitosis
E become coated with antibody on their surfaces

275
In an antigen-antibody reaction, macrophages
A may accumulate antigen on their surfaces
B secrete phytohaemagglutinin
C may be immobilised at the site of the reaction by a factor released from T lymphocytes
D become specifically cytostatic to cells bearing the antigen
E may act as scavengers of cells already damaged by T lymphocytes

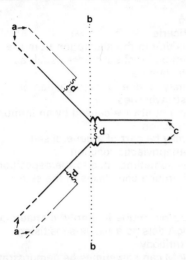

276
In the diagram of an immunoglobulin molecule above
A antigen-binding occurs at the sites labelled a

B reducing agents cause the molecule to break at the site labelled b

C the part of the molecule predominantly responsible for complement activation is labelled c

D the parts labelled d are called light chains

E the part of the molecule labelled c is responsible for the antigenic differences between the classes of immunoglobulins

277
Immunoglobulin
A G is the predominant immunoglobulin in normal serum

B A is largely manufactured in the laminae propriae of the respiratory and intestinal mucosa

C M is predominantly intravascular

D E is transported across the placenta

E D is especially effective in activating complement

278
The pathophysiological functions of the different classes of immunoglobulins are as follows:
A haemolysis : IgM

B neutralization of soluble toxin : IgG

C production of hayfever : IgD

D agglutination of bacteria : IgA

E protection against poliomyelitis : IgE

279
Severe combined immunodeficiency
A may present with tetany in the newborn

B can sometimes be diagnosed in fetal life

C is inherited as an autosomal dominant trait

D is a contra-indication to smallpox vaccination

E causes both lymphopenia and agammaglobulinaemia

280
X-linked recessive hypogammaglobulinaemia
A is compatible with survival for many years

B can be effectively treated with weekly injections of immunoglobulin

C causes increased susceptibility to fungal infection

D is associated with lymphopenia

E causes follicular hyperplasia in lymph nodes

281
In primary acquired agammaglobulinaemia
A the sex incidence is equal

B there is an unusually high incidence of pernicious anaemia

C Giardia lamblia infection is common

D chickenpox carries a high mortality

E cutaneous granulomas are a recognised feature

282
Failure of a patient's T lymphocytes to respond in vitro to phytohaemagglutinin by transformation to lymphoblasts is a recognised occurrence in
A sarcoidosis
B Wiskott-Aldrich syndrome
C uraemia
D prematurity
E Hodgkin's disease

283
The following statements are correct:
A Immune complex disease may result from complement deficiency
B Bence-Jones proteinuria is pathognomonic of multiple myeloma
C Heavy chains of IgG may rarely be present in the urine of patients with rapidly progressive lymphoma
D Multiple myeloma represents the malignant proliferation of a clone of T lymphocytes
E Patients with Waldenström's macroglobulinaemia are unusually resistant to bacterial infections

284
In Type I immune reactions in man
A the antibody is always IgE
B an antigen-antibody reaction occurs on the surface of mast cells
C most of the clinical manifestations are due to the release of kinins from mast cells
D anaphylaxis occurs only in atopic individuals
E bronchoconstriction may follow inhalation of reagin

285
The manifestations of systemic anaphylaxis include
A laryngeal oedema
B bronchospasm
C hypotension
D lymphadenopathy
E nausea and vomiting

286
Urticaria
A is due to the absorption from the intestine of substances such as histamine
B may be due to the ingestion of strawberries
C is not always caused by an immune reaction
D may be part of a generalised anaphylactic reaction
E is sometimes due to the deposition of immune complexes in the skin

287
In autoimmune haemolytic anaemia
A IgA acts as a tissue-sensitising antibody
B IgM can sometimes be demonstrated on the red cell surface
C haemolysis occurs if antihuman globulin is added to a suspension of the patient's red cells
D the immune reaction is Type II
E the damaged red cells are destroyed in the spleen or liver

288
Immune complexes
A with antibody excess are the most likely to react with complement
B with great antigen excess are the most likely to be deposited in vessel walls
C induce inflammation if they are of intermediate size and are soluble
D may be visible under the electron microscope
E become trapped in renal glomerular vessels only if the antigen is derived from glomerular basement membrane

289
Lesions due to immune complexes occur in
A infective endocarditis
B systemic lupus erythematosus
C Goodpasture's syndrome
D pernicious anaemia
E post-streptococcal proliferative glomerulo-nephritis

290
Type IV immune reactions are characteristically involved in
A lepromatous leprosy
B tuberculosis
C polyarteritis
D measles
E Hashimoto's thyroiditis

291
The evidence in favour of a rash being due to a Type IV immune reaction is as follows:
A The serum concentration of IgE is very high
B The skin lesions develop within a few minutes of exposure to an antigen
C Hypersensitivity to an antigen can be transferred to a normal subject by an injection of the patient's lymphocytes
D The patient's lymphocytes take up tritiated thymidine avidly
E Complement can be demonstrated in the lesions by an immunofluorescence technique

292
IgG antibodies play a part in the following immune reactions:
A Type I
B Type II
C Type III
D Type IV
E Type V

293
A Type VI immune reaction
A requires immune complexes to be produced in the presence of excess antigen to be effective
B requires complement for cell lysis to occur
C occurs in schistosomiasis
D is initiated through contact of a K cell with the Fab portion of an antibody molecule
E may sometimes be responsible for regression of a tumour

294
In auto-immune diseases
A the most important immune mechanism is Type I
B a micro-organism which shares an antigen with the patient's tissue may be responsible for initiating the process
C deterioration of the function of some T cells may be of aetiological importance
D auto-antibodies are formed continually over a period of years
E K cells play no part

295
Antihistamines
A act on the same tissue receptors as adrenaline
B are ineffective in bronchial asthma
C inhibit the effects of bradykinin as well as those of histamine
D reduce the manifestations of acute urticaria
E may produce tachycardia and palpitations

296
The following drugs are effective in the treatment of an acute attack of bronchial asthma:
A salbutamol
B disodium cromoglycate
C aminophylline
D salicylates
E hydrocortisone

297
The process of hyposensitisation
A involves the intravenous injection of antigen
B results in the production of IgG antibodies against the antigen
C carries some risk of causing a Type III immune reaction
D leads to blocking of the combination of IgE with the antigen
E can sometimes prevent the development of hayfever or asthma

298

Agents used for the treatment of undesirable effects of immune reactions act as follows:

A Antilymphocyte serum : reduction in antibody formation

B Azathioprine : interference with the division of lymphoid cells

C Corticosteroids : interference with the function of T lymphocytes

D Indomethacin : 'anti-inflammatory' effect

E Disodium cromoglycate : inhibition of histamine release

299

The side-effects of the administration of antilymphocyte serum include

A a Type I immune reaction

B the development of lymphomas

C a Type III immune reaction

D bone marrow suppression

E a Type IV immune reaction

CHAPTER THREE

300

The following infections are described as zoonoses:

A leptospirosis

B brucellosis

C salmonellosis

D blastomycosis

E typhoid fever

301

The following diseases are typically spread by the ingestion of infected water or food:

A cholera

B poliomyelitis

C Weil's disease

D Virus B hepatitis

E bacillary dysentery

302

The following statements are correct:

A Meningococcal infection is mainly disseminated by the faecal-oral route

B A commensal organism living on the surface of the skin does not cause disease in any circumstances

C The term fomites is restricted to inanimate articles

D The incubation periods of bacterial diseases range from a few days to several years

E Urinary infections may arise from an autogenous source

303

Useful evidence about the nature or site of an infection may be provided by

A a history of residence abroad

B knowledge of the patient's occupation

C a history of alcoholism

D the presence of diabetes mellitus

E a history of a recent laparotomy

304

Direct microscopy of an appropriately prepared specimen is useful in the diagnosis of

A pulmonary tuberculosis

B gonorrhoea

C brucellosis

D primary syphilis

E mumps

305
Estimation of specific antibodies in serum
A is of value in the diagnosis of brucellosis
B is most useful when carried out very early in the course of the illness
C is of particular value if the test is repeated after 5–7 days
D yields results of which the interpretation may be influenced by previous artificial immunisation
E is generally of greater immediate value in viral than in bacterial infections

306
In the investigation of a case of pyrexia of unknown origin
A radiography is rarely of value
B modification of the patient's treatment may be of diagnostic value
C rubella is an important cause in children
D Hodgkin's disease should be suspected if the skin is cool despite high fever
E study of the temperature chart may be helpful

307
The following measures are of value in the prevention of spread of the diseases named:
A use of insecticides—malaria
B quarantine—smallpox
C isolation of the patient—infective endocarditis
D topical penicillin in soaps and creams—autogenous infections
E active immunisation—yellow fever

308
The schedule of immunisation generally followed in the United Kingdom includes
A five doses of oral poliomyelitis vaccine
B measles vaccination in the first year followed by a booster at the age of 10–13
C rubella vaccination for girls aged 11–13
D influenza vaccination on leaving school
E BCG for the tuberculin-negative at 10–13 years

309
Scarlet fever
A should not be diagnosed unless severe tonsillitis is present
B cannot be diagnosed in the absence of the rash
C has an incubation period of 10–14 days
D is a notifiable disease
E is associated with generalised lymphadenopathy

310
The rash of scarlet fever
A usually appears first behind the ears
B is typically profuse on the face
C is succeeded by desquamation of the skin
D is due to a specific streptococcal exotoxin
E is commonly intense on the flexures of the arms and legs

311
Erysipelas
A is commoner in young people than in the elderly
B is painful
C characteristically spares the region around the mouth if the face is affected
D is associated with clearly defined patches of inflamed skin
E should be treated with penicillin

312
Staphylococcus pyogenes
A has been undergoing a spontaneous decline in virulence for several years
B is almost always resistant to benzylpenicillin
C is a recognised cause of food poisoning
D characteristically causes suppuration
E can be isolated from the skin or nasopharynx of up to 30 per cent of healthy persons

313

In whooping-cough

A the characteristic whoop is usually first heard 14–21 days after exposure to the infection

B the cough is unproductive throughout the illness

C infectivity is at its highest when the whoop is most prominent

D the cough is typically accompanied by vomiting

E segmental pulmonary collapse is a recognised complication

314

Upper respiratory catarrh is the most common presenting symptom in

A diphtheria

B chickenpox

C rubella

D measles

E whooping-cough

315

Features of diphtheria which are of value in distinguishing it from streptococcal tonsillitis include

A firmly adherent membrane on the tonsils

B cervical lymphadenopathy

C high fever

D spread of the exudate beyond the tonsils

E paralysis of the palate

316

Complications of diphtheria include

A acute laryngeal obstruction

B cardiac failure

C permanent respiratory paralysis

D acute otitis media

E paralysis of accommodation

317

In the treatment of diphtheria

A antitoxin should rarely be given until the diagnosis has been confirmed bacteriologically

B serum sickness from administration of antitoxin does not occur if the patient has never previously received horse serum

C complete rest is essential for at least three weeks

D the patient should be isolated until the membrane has disappeared

E the antibiotic of choice is penicillin

318

During the first week of an attack of typhoid fever

A the organisms are more likely to be isolated from the stools than from the blood

B constipation is more common than diarrhoea

C haemorrhage from the bowel is unusual

D the Widal reaction is unlikely to be of diagnostic value

E the typical rash appears and rapidly fades

319

Paratyphoid fever

A is less likely to cause a rash than typhoid

B often presents with acute enteritis

C should be treated with co-trimoxazole

D has an incubation period of 14–21 days

E is usually transmitted by the faecal-oral route

320

The evening after a lunch party at which meat pie and chips were eaten some of the diners complain of abdominal pain and vomiting and, later, diarrhoea

A Contamination of the food by a chemical poison is a likely cause

B Salmonella food poisoning is less likely than staphylococcal

C The vomiting is more in favour of *Cl. welchii* than of staphylococcal food poisoning

D Blood and pus are likely to be present in the stools

E All the diners, whether affected or not, should be given ampicillin

321
The incidence of bacterial food poisoning can be reduced by
A an increased consumption of battery-reared poultry
B keeping cooked meat in a refrigerator
C cooking poultry as soon as possible after it has been removed from a deep freeze
D using hen's rather than duck's eggs for making custard
E keeping cooked food in glass rather than enamel containers

322
Bacillary dysentery
A in Britain is most often due to *Shigella sonnei*
B is characterised by profuse watery diarrhoea
C is usually a febrile illness
D has a more acute onset than amoebic dysentery
E is most commonly spread by contamination of the water supply with sewage

323
Characteristic features of tetanus include
A painful spasm of the masseter muscles
B abdominal rigidity without tenderness
C loss of consciousness during the convulsions
D lymphocytosis in the cerebrospinal fluid
E an incubation period of 2–3 days

324
A patient with a heavily contaminated wound of the leg develops tetanus. The treatment should include
A the intravenous injection of tetanus antitoxin an hour or two after surgical removal of necrotic tissue from the wound
B the administration of cloxacillin
C the avoidance of intravenous feeding as this may provoke spasms
D prevention of spasms by diazepam
E as little disturbance of the patient as possible

325
Recognised features of brucellosis include
A splenomegaly
B sweating
C continuous fever
D neutrophil leucocytosis
E arthritis

326
Acute meningococcal infections are
A spread by the airborne route
B characterised by a maculopapular rash
C best treated with sulphadimidine
D associated with lymphocytosis in the peripheral blood
E sometimes complicated by disseminated intravascular coagulation

327
Gonorrhoea
A can cause blindness in infants
B is more likely to be asymptomatic in males than in females
C is the commonest cause of urethritis in males in Britain
D can be effectively treated with spectinomycin in patients allergic to penicillin
E should not be treated with penicillin until coexistent syphilis has been excluded

328
Recognised features of secondary syphilis include
A an itchy polymorphic rash
B generalised painless lymphadenopathy
C shallow ulcers on the buccal mucous membrane
D cranial nerve palsies
E gumma formation in the skin and subcutaneous tissues

329
In a patient with systemic lupus erythematosus co-existent syphilis can be confidently diagnosed if the following tests are positive:
A Venereal Disease Reference Laboratory (VDRL)
B Kahn
C Treponemal Immobilisation (TPI)
D Wassermann (WR)
E Fluorescent Treponemal Antibody (FTA)

330
In Weil's disease
A two separate episodes of pyrexia are to be expected
B jaundice is unlikely to develop until leptospiral antibodies appear in the blood
C the overall mortality is 15–20 per cent
D acute renal failure is a recognised cause of death
E a relapse with an exacerbation of jaundice is a recognised feature of the convalescent phase

331
Expected findings in leptospirosis include
A polymorphonuclear leucocytosis
B high protein concentration in the cerebrospinal fluid
C neck stiffness
D conjunctival suffusion
E isolation of the organism from the urine two weeks after the onset of the disease

332
The rash of measles
A is lighter in colour than that of rubella
B first appears behind the ears
C is preceded by swelling of the eyelids and lacrimation
D is accompanied by posterior cervical lymphadenopathy
E is preceded by Koplik's spots on the buccal mucosa

333
Recognised complications of measles include
A myocarditis
B otitis media
C pneumonia
D pancreatitis
E corneal ulceration

334
Rubella occurring in the first trimester of pregnancy
A is a recognised cause of deafness in the neonate
B is more likely to cause polyarthritis than in a child
C is an indication for termination of pregnancy
D is not uncommon even in women who have had the disease
E lasts for two or three days only

335
Mumps
A is less infectious than measles
B is complicated by orchitis in about 25 per cent of pre-pubertal male patients
C may present as acute meningitis
D is sometimes complicated by uveitis
E can cause difficulty in opening the mouth

336
Chickenpox is usually a mild disease except in patients
A in whom the lesions become pustular
B with leukaemia
C on corticosteroids
D who develop chickenpox pneumonia
E who become infected by a patient with herpes zoster

337
In variola minor
A the incubation period is over three weeks
B the distribution of the rash is similar to that in variola major
C the immunity which develops is less permanent than that resulting from vaccination
D the rash is usually sparse
E the prodromal illness is mild

338
Characteristic features of the rash of chickenpox include
A circular vesicles
B lesions at all stages of development present at the same time
C more profuse lesions on the forearms than on the shoulders
D sparing of the axillae
E evolution of individual lesions from macule to pustule in 24 hours

339
Contra-indications to vaccination against smallpox include
A infantile eczema
B pregnancy
C corticosteroid therapy
D leukaemia
E previous vaccination

340
The following antimicrobial agents are bactericidal:
A sulphadimidine
B flucloxacillin
C streptomycin
D oxytetracycline
E co-trimoxazole

341
The following antibiotics are effective against *Ps. aeruginosa*:
A cephalexin
B erythromycin
C carbenicillin
D gentamicin
E colistin (polymyxin E)

342
Adverse effects of sulphadimidine include
A agranulocytosis
B erythema multiforme
C megaloblastic anaemia
D haematuria
E haemolytic anaemia

343
Benzylpenicillin
A is unsuitable for intravenous injection
B is inactivated by staphylococcal penicillinase
C is destroyed by gastric acid
D diffuses freely into the cerebrospinal fluid
E causes skin rashes in over 90 per cent of patients with glandular fever

344
The following antibiotics are effective in systemic infections when given by mouth:
A gentamicin
B ampicillin
C cephaloridine
D amphotericin B
E cephalexin

345
Renal damage is a recognised adverse effect of
A tetracycline
B colistin (polymyxin E)
C streptomycin
D chloramphenicol
E cephaloridine

346
The tetracyclines are the antibiotics of choice in
A H. influenzae meningitis
B typhus fevers
C mycoplasma pneumonia
D Q fever
E lymphogranuloma venereum

347
Staphylococcal osteomyelitis will usually respond satisfactorily to treatment with
A streptomycin
B flucloxacillin
C clindamycin
D amoxycillin
E sodium fusidate

348
The following statements are correct:
A All the aminoglycoside antibiotics are effective in tuberculosis
B The lincomycins are effective against *Bacteroides* infections
C Fatal pancytopenia is a recognised adverse effect of chloramphenicol
D Erythromycin can cause severe liver damage
E Nitrofurantoin is indicated only for urinary tract infections

349
There are special hazards involved in the administration to neonates of
A nalidixic acid
B erythromycin
C nitrofurantoin
D chloramphenicol
E tetracycline

350
Antimicrobial agents effective against fungi include
A idoxuridine
B nystatin
C amphotericin B
D amikacin
E cytarabine

351
It is usually correct clinical practice to administer an appropriate antibiotic on the basis of clinical findings in
A bacillary dysentery
B staphylococcal osteomyelitis
C follicular tonsillitis
D an acute exacerbation of chronic bronchitis
E lobar pneumonia

352
Clinical situations exist in which the following drug combinations are rational therapy:
A kanamycin and gentamicin
B ampicillin and cloxacillin
C cephaloridine and frusemide
D benzylpenicillin and probenecid
E benzylpenicillin and streptomycin

CHAPTER FOUR

353
Undernutrition
A is due to a qualitative dietary deficiency
B and malnutrition may both be due to renal failure
C is an important feature of chronic alcoholism
D is a recognised cause of diarrhoea
E is an inevitable consequence of a strict vegetarian diet

354
In spite of a satisfactory and balanced diet, the following conditions can lead to the nutritional disorders stated:
A achlorhydria—protein deficiency due to impaired digestion
B chronic alcoholism—Wernicke's encephalopathy
C hepatic cirrhosis—vitamin A deficiency
D Hartnup disease—scurvy
E epilepsy treated with phenytoin—osteomalacia

355
Good health can be maintained by a moderately active man on a diet containing
A enough food to provide 1700 kcal per day
B no cystine
C 50 g of carbohydrate per day
D 60 g of animal protein per day
E 15mg of iron per day

356
Recognised features of starvation include
A nocturnal polyuria
B raised haematocrit value
C intestinal lactase deficiency
D cardiac enlargement
E increasing oedema on re-feeding unless salt is restricted

357
The following statements are correct:
A Starch, sucrose or glucose are essential elements in the diet because the body cannot synthesise glucose
B Fats provide the greater part of the energy content of a normal diet
C Essential fatty acids are required for the synthesis of prostaglandins
D One or more essential amino-acids are deficient in most vegetable proteins
E Protein of high biological value is provided by a mixture of cereals and legumes

358
Protein-calorie malnutrition
A is a term which includes a variety of forms of malnutrition
B is the commonest dietary deficiency disease in the world
C means that the calorific value of the diet is inadequate due to a shortage of protein
D is invariably characterised by a severe weight deficit in relation to the child's height
E may produce a clinical picture resembling that due to abdominal tuberculosis

359
Recognised features of kwashiorkor in a child include
A liver enlargement due to fatty change
B ascites which is disproportionately more severe than the degree of peripheral oedema present
C maintenance of lively mental and physical activity
D pigmentary changes in the hair
E skin changes simulating pellagra

360
During the treatment of kwashiorkor
A an immediate fall in the child's weight suggests that an associated condition such as abdominal tuberculosis should be considered
B there is a risk of hyperpyrexia
C feeding with animal protein is essential
D potassium chloride should be given orally
E intestinal lactase deficiency should be treated by giving ample amounts of milk in the diet

361
Kwashiorkor
A is commonly precipitated by malaria
B has a mortality of around 20 per cent in the early days of treatment
C is complicated by anaemia which is usually megaloblastic
D frequently leads to cirrhosis of the liver in adult life
E can be prevented by modification of local agricultural practice

362
Nutritional marasmus
A in contrast to kwashiorkor, usually affects urban children
B affects particularly 3 to 4 year old children
C is principally due to late weaning
D presents with both retardation of growth and reduction of weight
E is typically associated with the passage of watery or semi-solid, bulky, acid stools

363
Protein-calorie malnutrition
A may be diagnosed in the 'prekwashiorkor' stage by finding characteristic biochemical abnormalities
B in a mild or moderate form affects up to 50 per cent of children under 5 in some countries
C is probably the main cause of the very high mortality of 1–4 year old children in developing countries
D can be detected early by comparing a child's weight with the normal international standard for his age
E is likely to become less common as urbanisation proceeds in developing countries

364
Deficiency of
A phosphorus is unlikely in the absence of calcium deficiency
B zinc is of no known significance
C iodine is a recognised cause of goitre
D fluorine causes sclerosis of bone and calcification of ligaments
E copper impairs the action of insulin

C

365
The intestinal absorption of calcium
A is enhanced if phytic acid is added to bread
B is normally incomplete as 75 per cent of ingested calcium is excreted in the faeces
C is less efficient in children in tropical countries
D is impaired if it is ingested together with spinach
E from vegetables and cereals is a significant contribution to the total absorption

366
The following statements are correct:
A The fluoridation of water has little effect on the teeth of adults
B Excessive fluorine in water can cause mottling of the teeth
C Phosphate depletion may result from excessive intake of magnesium trisilicate
D In the United Kingdom manufacturers are legally required to add iodine to table salt
E Siderosis with hepatic cirrhosis is a recognised consequence of the excessive ingestion of iron

367
Vitamin deficiencies due to factors other than an inadequate diet include deficiency of
A folate due to phenytoin therapy
B vitamin A due to an antivitamin in raw fish
C hydroxocobalamin due to bacterial colonisation of the small intestine
D vitamin K_1 due to sterilisation of the bowel with neomycin
E vitamin C due to malabsorption of fat

368
Vitamin A
A deficiency is one of the commonest causes of blindness in the world
B is present in high concentration in olive oil
C is stored in large quantities in the human liver
D deficiency causes a disturbance of vision similar to that of retinitis pigmentosa
E deficiency causes profuse watering of the eyes in the earliest stage of xerophthalmia

369
Vitamin D
A is formed by ultraviolet irradiation of ergosterol in the skin
B is stored in large amounts in the human liver
C is synthesised better in the skin of black races because of the more efficient absorption of light
D stimulates the synthesis of a calcium transport protein in the mucosa of the small intestine
E is hydroxylated in the liver and kidney to 1,25 dihydrocholecalciferol

370
Rickets
A affects an older age group in Britain than it does in developing countries
B cannot be diagnosed in the absence of hypocalcaemia or hypophosphataemia
C is characterised by a rise in the serum alkaline phosphatase activity
D in British Asian children arises solely because of peculiarities in their diet
E is associated with a tendency to overactivity of the parathyroids

371
Recognised clinical features of vitamin D deficiency in children include
A delay in the normal stages of development
B a scaphoid abdomen
C broadening of the distal end of the radius
D hypotonia
E tetany

372
When treating a child with rickets
A a daily dose of 10μg of vitamin D is sufficient
B there is usually no need to give additional calcium if sufficient vitamin D is given
C biochemical changes are more reliable than radiography in assessing the rate of recovery
D failure to respond to ordinary therapeutic doses of vitamin D may be due to chronic renal failure
E overdosage with vitamin D may cause renal failure

373
Recognised features of osteomalacia include
A biconcave upper and lower borders of the vertebral bodies
B skeletal pain
C symmetrical translucent bands on the axillary borders of the scapulae
D muscular weakness
E a tendency to spontaneous improvement

374
Osteoporosis
A is commoner in women than in men
B may be partly caused by a low protein diet
C is a recognised feature of Cushing's syndrome
D usually causes no symptoms
E may be due to a previous partial gastrectomy

375
In osteoporosis the
A amount of osteoid in the bones is normal
B development of the disease is delayed by rest
C healing of fractures is impaired
D serum alkaline phosphatase activity is raised
E best treatment for vertebral collapse is a spinal support

376
Ascorbic acid
A is required for the formation of collagen
B may be destroyed if food is badly cooked
C is in low concentration in leucocytes but not in plasma in clinical scurvy
D is rapidly excreted in the urine after an oral dose
E has no known toxic effects even in very large doses

377
In scurvy
A in children osteomyelitis may be simulated
B the characteristic gum changes are most severe in the edentulous
C the patient is usually anaemic
D bleeding is most prominent in the upper limbs
E wound healing is impaired

378
Deficiency of thiamin
A causes defective DNA synthesis
B causes accumulation of lactate and pyruvate
C is less likely to occur if the diet is rich in carbohydrate
D can cause an increase in cardiac output
E is more likely to occur if the diet consists largely of tinned foods

379
Recognised features of beriberi include
A 'woody legs'
B follicular keratosis
C pain in the legs on walking
D raised jugular venous pressure
E sluggish tendon jerks

380
Characteristic features of Wernicke's encephalopathy include
A nystagmus
B papilloedema
C reduced red cell transketolase activity
D confabulation
E delusions

381
Intramuscular administration of thiamin can produce improvement in the following manifestations of thiamin deficiency within a few hours:
A dyspnoea
B ophthalmoplegia
C paraesthesiae
D impairment of memory
E muscular tenderness

382
Pellagra
A is exceptional in countries where maize is the staple cereal
B is a recognised cause of a red swollen tongue
C is a cause of light-sensitive dermatitis
D may be manifest only by dementia in women in purdah
E must be treated with nicotinamide for many weeks before improvement can be expected

383
The rash of pellagra
A is symmetrical
B affects the face and neck particularly
C is dry and scaly in chronic cases
D is usually the first manifestation of the disease
E does not affect moist areas such as the perineum

384
The clinical features of riboflavin deficiency in man include
A angular stomatitis
B amblyopia
C diarrhoea
D naso-labial seborrhoea
E convulsions

385
Vitamin B$_{12}$ deficiency
A can result from a strict vegetarian diet
B occurs in Addisonian pernicious anaemia because intrinsic factor protects the vitamin from destruction by gastric acid
C is not evident for at least four years after total gastrectomy
D can cause neuropathy without significant anaemia
E may complicate haemolytic anaemias

386
Obesity
A is the commonest nutritional disorder of affluent societies
B is commoner in the children of obese than in those of lean parents
C is a term used to describe gain in weight from any cause
D may be the cause of a psychological disturbance
E is usefully assessed by measurement of skin-fold thickness over the triceps

387
Recognised causes of obesity include
A emotional deprivation
B diabetes mellitus
C the habit of taking frequent small meals rather than one large meal daily
D Cushing's syndrome
E the high cost of less fattening foods

388
The following statements about obesity are correct:
A Physical activity is greater in lean people than in the obese
B Energy expenditure for a given amount of exercise is less in the obese
C Women are more often affected than men
D Loss of weight after the menopause commonly corrects obesity which developed in earlier years
E Insulin promotes lipogenesis and inhibits lipolysis

389
Recognised complications of obesity include
A osteoarthrosis
B renal calculi
C varicose veins
D intertrigo
E angina pectoris

390
In the treatment of obesity
A a diet of about 1000 kcal (4200 kJ)/day is usually satisfactory
B regular daily exercise should be taken
C a diet of 400 kcal (1680 kJ)/day must be accompanied by strict rest
D amphetamines can be prescribed for a few months at a time
E regular doses of thyroxine are valuable in resistant cases even in the absence of hypothyroidism

CHAPTER FIVE

391
The following statements are correct:
A The volumes of intracellular and extracellular water are about equal
B Most of the extracellular water is in the interstitial fluid
C The osmotic pressure is normally identical in intracellular and extracellular fluids
D The extracellular fluid concentration of magnesium is approximately 1 mmol/l
E The hydrogen ion concentration of extracellular fluid is about 40 mmol/l

392
The following ions are present in higher concentration in the extracellular than in the intracellular fluid:
A chloride
B potassium
C phosphate
D bicarbonate
E hydrogen

393
Sodium depletion
A is usually the result of excessive loss of salt rather than inadequate intake
B is usually accompanied by a corresponding reduction in the water content of the body
C is a recognised feature of the diuretic phase of acute tubular necrosis of ischaemic origin
D is exceptional in diabetic ketoacidosis
E is a characteristic complication of cystic disease of the pancreas

394
Characteristic consequences of predominant sodium depletion include
A thirst
B hypotension
C uraemia
D loss of skin elasticity
E bradycardia

395
During the treatment of sodium depletion
A intravenous dextrose is contraindicated
B the lung bases should be examined frequently
C intravenous isotonic sodium chloride solution is not indicated unless the plasma sodium concentration is below normal
D disturbance of potassium balance may also need correction
E the best guides to the amount of salt needed are the responses of the blood pressure and pulse rate

396
Primary water depletion
A is associated with a reduction in the amount of water lost from the body in the expired air and by evaporation from the skin
B is more common in clinical practice than sodium depletion
C is a recognised complication of hyperparathyroidism
D is characteristically associated with signs of gross dehydration
E is best treated by intravenous infusion of isotonic sodium chloride

397
Recognised causes of potassium depletion include
A Cushing's syndrome
B administration of carbenoxolone
C metabolic alkalosis
D the administration of spironolactone
E heart failure

398
The following statements regarding potassium depletion are correct:
A The normal daily intake of potassium is about 8–10 g
B Significant depletion of potassium may occur without alteration of the plasma potassium concentration
C In potassium depletion the plasma bicarbonate concentration is characteristically reduced
D Intravenous infusion of potassium is best avoided in the presence of oliguria
E Prophylactic oral potassium chloride should be given to patients being treated with corticosteroids

399
Recognised consequences of potassium depletion include
A polyuria
B reduced sensitivity to digitalis
C tall T waves in the electrocardiogram
D a diminution in the plasma sodium concentration
E muscular spasticity

400
Potassium excess
A is a recognised feature of Addisonian crisis
B is a recognised association of severe oliguria
C can be distinguished from potassium depletion by the flaccidity of the paralysis it produces
D is a recognised cause of atrioventricular conduction defects
E carries a risk of cardiac arrest if the plasma potassium concentration exceeds 7.5 mmol/l

401
The following measures are of value in the treatment of potassium excess:
A fruit juices given orally
B correction of water and salt depletion
C oral administration of a sodium loaded ionic exchange resin
D the administration of subcutaneous insulin and oral glucose
E peritoneal dialysis

402
Magnesium deficiency
A is a recognised feature of kwashiorkor
B is a characteristic feature of hypoparathyroidism
C is a recognised finding in chronic alcoholism
D may cause epileptiform convulsions
E is best treated by oral magnesium supplements

403
Impaired ability to dilute the urine when large amounts of water are given is a recognised feature of
A adrenocortical overactivity
B hepatic cirrhosis
C chronic renal disease
D the post-operative state
E severe heart failure

404
Retention of sodium is a recognised consequence of the administration of
A carbenoxolone
B oestrogen-containing oral contraceptives
C thiamin
D triamterene
E phenylbutazone

405
Regarding diuretics,
A frusemide is a benzothiadiazine derivative
B hyperuricaemia is a recognised complication of bendrofluazide therapy
C the predominant action of ethacrynic acid is to reduce the reabsorption of sodium and chloride in the ascending limb of the loop of Henle
D hypokalaemia is a recognised consequence of triamterene therapy
E amiloride exerts its effects by competing for aldosterone combining sites

406
Chronic diarrhoea is a recognised cause of
A sodium depletion
B magnesium deficiency
C water intoxication
D potassium depletion
E metabolic alkalosis

407
Diuretic-induced sodium depletion
A is less likely to occur in the treatment of ascites if repeated abdominal paracenteses are performed
B cannot occur if the patient remains oedematous
C is characterised by mental apathy
D is less likely to occur with the use of frusemide than with benzothiadiazine diuretics
E may be relieved symptomatically by intravenous infusion of hypertonic saline

408
The following statements regarding the regulation of hydrogen ion concentration are correct:
A Plasma proteins are quite strong acids
B The pH of the blood depends principally upon the ratio of carbonic acid and bicarbonate
C Chloride ions enter the red cells in the pulmonary capillaries
D The concentration of bicarbonate in the plasma is regulated by the partial pressure of carbon dioxide in the alveoli
E A proportion of carbon dioxide is transported in the blood reversibly bound to haemoglobin

409
Carbonic acid
A is produced by metabolic reactions in normal man in smaller amounts than is acetoacetic acid
B is buffered in the red blood cell by haemoglobin
C appears in the blood predominantly as bicarbonate ion
D together with carbon dioxide forms an important buffer system in the blood
E if present in excess in the body is removed by the kidneys

410
In the investigation of disturbances in hydrogen ion concentration
A the concentration of bicarbonate ion in plasma is a more valid measurement of acidity than is the blood pH
B 'standard bicarbonate' refers to the concentration of bicarbonate ion in a plasma sample which would exist at a standard $PaCO_2$ value of 5.3 kPa
C in conventional laboratory practice, blood pH is calculated from a knowledge of $PaCO_2$ and bicarbonate ion concentration
D the normal pH of plasma is about 7.2
E estimation of urinary ammonium concentration is to some extent a measure of hydrogen ion excretion

411
Metabolic acidosis
A is characterised by a rise in the plasma bicarbonate concentration
B is typically associated with a reduced $PaCO_2$
C occurs most commonly as a result of vigorous exercise
D in chronic renal failure is due in part to diminished secretion of hydrogen and ammonium ions by the kidneys
E occurring as a complication of acetazolamide administration is due to increased formation of carbonic acid in the red cell

412
The following statements are correct:
A The acid-base disturbance in chronic diarrhoea is due to direct loss of bicarbonate in the stools
B Provided renal function is normal, administration of isotonic saline is usually effective in correcting mild metabolic acidosis
C Potassium depletion is a recognised cause of metabolic acidosis
D Chloride deficiency leads to metabolic alkalosis by preventing the operation of the chloride shift between plasma and red cells
E The effect of a lowered hydrogen ion concentration in the blood is mitigated by an increase in the ionisation of blood carbonic acid

413
Recognised associations of metabolic alkalosis due to prolonged vomiting include
A secretion of urine of acid pH
B delirium
C tetany
D proteinuria
E a rise in $PaCO_2$

CHAPTER SIX

414
The following statements are correct:
A Sudden attacks of nocturnal dyspnoea may be the presenting feature of left heart failure
B The distribution of oedema in heart failure is mainly determined by gravity
C Exercise syncope is usually not due to heart disease
D In heart failure epigastric pain may result from distension of the liver
E Palpitation means an awareness that the heart beats are irregular

415
Syncope
A is more often due to heart disease than to any other single cause
B may be preceded by failure of vision
C is characterised by bradycardia
D can be indirectly due to retention of urine
E can be due to venous pooling in dependent parts

416
The following statements about the arterial pulse are correct:
A Raising the arm increases the 'knocking' quality of the pulse in aortic regurgitation
B A small volume pulse is characteristic of complete heart block
C An anacrotic pulse is typical of aortic stenosis
D A small stroke volume produces a small volume pulse
E Diminished arterial pulsation in the neck is characteristic of coarctation of the aorta

417
In the jugular venous pulse
A the pulse waves disappear in the presence of a large pericardial effusion
B the pressure rises after a large pulmonary embolism
C a prominent 'a' wave is seen in the presence of superior vena caval obstruction
D the 'y' descent is synchronous with the end of atrial contraction
E the 'x' descent is absent in severe tricuspid regurgitation

418
The following signs provide reliable diagnostic evidence of the disorders listed with them:
A an apex beat lateral to the mid-clavicular line—cardiac enlargement
B an abnormally forceful apical impulse—aortic stenosis
C an apical diastolic thrill—mitral stenosis
D pulsation to the left of the sternum—right ventricular hypertrophy
E a systolic thrill at the lower left sternal edge—tricuspid regurgitation

419
The following statements about auscultation of the heart are correct:
A The diaphragm of the stethoscope applied lightly favours the transmission of low-pitched sounds and murmurs
B An abnormally quiet first sound may be due to ischaemic damage to papillary muscles
C Accentuation of the apical first sound may be caused by anxiety
D The second sound is accentuated in calcific aortic stenosis
E Reversed splitting of the second sound is a feature of pulmonary hypertension

420
On auscultation of the heart
A in a normal child a low-pitched fourth sound is often heard at the apex
B a fourth sound is comparable in its genesis to the 'a' wave of the venous pulse
C the opening snap of mitral stenosis is best heard at the apex
D the murmur of semilunar valve regurgitation is typically harsh and saw-like
E in an adult a fourth sound is a feature of longstanding arterial hypertension

421
The following statements about electrocardiography are correct:
A A potassium ion gradient is mainly responsible for the electrical potential difference across the cell membrane
B Only one electrode is connected to the galvanometer to record a V lead
C An exploring electrode records an upward deflection when the depolarisation current is flowing away from it
D The amplitude of the QRS complex is related to the bulk of muscle tissue through which the impulse is passing
E The T wave is due to ventricular repolarisation

422
In a normal electrocardiogram
A the P wave is due to activity of the sino-atrial node
B the initial deflection of the QRS complex is upwards in lead V1
C the R wave is larger than the S wave in lead V1
D the T wave is upright in lead aVR
E a Q wave is present in lead V6

423
In the investigation of a patient with heart disease
A the chest X-ray is unlikely to show evidence of pulmonary oedema if there are no abnormal physical signs in the chest
B displacement of the barium-filled oesophagus in a chest X-ray is evidence of left atrial enlargement
C an echocardiogram is easier to record if the lungs are overinflated as in emphysema
D the left atrial pressure cannot be measured except by left atrial puncture
E phonocardiography is required to distinguish the murmur of pulmonary regurgitation from that of aortic regurgitation

424
Measurement of intravascular pressures by catheterisation is of diagnostic value in
A aortic stenosis
B persistent ductus arteriosus
C atrial septal defect
D pulmonary stenosis
E ventricular septal defect

425
In sinus rhythm
A the heart rate is faster during inspiration than expiration
B the heart rate is never so slow as to cause syncope
C tachycardia may be due to re-entry
D athletes and patients with hyperthyroidism have similar heart rates
E the heart rate rarely exceeds 160/min in adults

426
In paroxysmal atrial tachycardia
A dropped beats may be felt in the radial pulse
B the heart is usually otherwise normal
C the attacks may be terminated by carotid sinus massage
D the attacks are typically followed by oliguria
E overindulgence in tobacco is known to precipitate attacks

427
Paroxysmal atrial tachycardia with atrio-ventricular block
A is associated with a ventricular rate of 140-220/min
B can be restored to sinus rhythm with intravenous practolol
C seldom occurs in otherwise normal hearts
D can be due to digitalis intoxication
E can sometimes be effectively treated with digoxin

428
In atrial flutter
A the arterial pulse is usually regular
B carotid sinus massage causes the pulse to become irregular
C the commonest underlying disorder in the elderly is ischaemic heart disease
D digoxin can convert the rhythm to atrial fibrillation
E the electrocardiogram shows F waves at a rate of about 20/sec

429
If a patient with mitral stenosis develops atrial fibrillation
A the left atrial pressure rises
B sinus rhythm should be restored with DC shock before advising valvotomy
C no f waves will be present in the electrocardiogram until several months have passed
D the presystolic murmur disappears
E the risk of embolism is greatest during the next few days

430
Ventricular extrasystoles
A are good evidence of ischaemic heart disease
B cannot be distinguished from atrial extrasystoles in the arterial pulse
C can precipitate ventricular fibrillation after myocardial infarction if they are unusually premature
D may cause heart failure
E may result from digoxin overdosage

431
Cardiac arrest
A is more often due to ventricular fibrillation than to asystole
B causes deep respiration due to the associated acidosis
C causes irreversible brain damage if the circulation cannot be restored within 30 seconds
D is easier to treat if it is due to asystole rather than to ventricular fibrillation
E should be diagnosed only if no pulse can be felt in a large artery

432
The treatment of cardiac arrest includes
A defibrillation once a definite diagnosis of ventricular fibrillation has been made from the electrocardiogram
B elevation of the legs
C intravenous digoxin
D intravenous sodium bicarbonate
E external massage applied to the region of the manubrium sterni

433
The following statements about heart block are correct:
A First degree atrioventricular block cannot be distinguished from sino-atrial block without an electrocardiogram
B Wenckebach's phenomenon is a dropped beat following progressive lengthening of successive P-R intervals
C 3 : 2 atrioventricular block can be distinguished from ectopic beats by auscultation
D Right bundle branch block may be a benign congenital condition
E In complete atrioventricular block the atrial rate is usually less than 40 per minute

434
Drugs which may be indicated in the long-term prophylaxis of ventricular tachycardia include
A quinidine
B mexiletine
C lignocaine
D practolol
E procainamide

435
Digoxin
A is indicated in the majority of patients with atrial fibrillation
B can convert atrial flutter to sinus rhythm
C acts mainly on the myocardial cell membrane
D can cause arrhythmias for which phenytoin is particularly effective treatment
E can be used to prevent paroxysmal atrial tachycardia

436
Following a severe haemorrhage
A the patient should be kept cool to discourage sweating
B metaraminol is indicated to raise the blood pressure
C a fall in central venous pressure suggests that blood transfusion has been too rapid
D acidosis is a possible complication
E bradycardia is more likely than tachycardia

437
Dilatation of
A both ventricles is a feature of severe anaemia
B the right ventricle occurs with an atrial septal defect
C a ventricle causes it to perform more work for a given cardiac output
D the left ventricle occurs in mitral stenosis
E both ventricles occurs in the presence of a pericardial effusion

438
In cardiac failure
A the reduced glomerular filtration rate is an important cause of sodium retention
B oversecretion of anti-diuretic hormone is the main endocrine factor causing fluid retention
C potassium retention occurs unless diuretics are administered
D the speed of development of the causative lesion is an important determinant of the clinical manifestations
E aldosterone antagonists are a very effective means of removing oedema

439
The following statements are correct:
A The onset of atrial fibrillation in mitral stenosis may precipitate pulmonary oedema
B Tricuspid regurgitation is almost exclusively of rheumatic origin
C Dilatation of the lower lobe pulmonary veins is the most reliable radiographic evidence of left atrial hypertension
D Cardiac failure due to aortic stenosis may become irreversible as a result of myocardial fibrosis
E Cachexia is a recognised consequence of chronic cardiac failure

440
In the treatment of severe cardiac failure
A regular exercise should be advised to maintain the circulation
B the patient should be allowed to sit out of bed only when dyspnoea has been relieved
C frusemide should be given last thing at night to prevent nocturnal dyspnoea
D moderate salt restriction should be advised
E hyponatraemia with persistent oedema suggests that the total body sodium is dangerously low and diuretics should be withheld

441
Toxic effects of digoxin
A are more likely to occur in the elderly
B are unlikely to occur unless the blood level exceeds 5 mg/100 ml
C may be aggravated by the concomitant administration of beta receptor blocking drugs
D include hypokalaemia
E are unlikely to occur in an adult on a daily dose of 0.125 mg

442
Recognised features of acute rheumatic fever include
A the development of a high degree of immunity to further attacks
B acute polyarthritis affecting particularly the proximal interphalangeal joints
C erythema marginatum
D prolongation of the P-R interval in the electrocardiogram
E a rising agglutination titre to *Streptococcus viridans*

443
Rheumatic nodules
A are painful
B tend to occur over the elbows and knees
C are commoner in adults than in children
D rarely occur unless active carditis is present
E are attached to the skin

444
In a patient with acute rheumatic fever
A rest in bed is necessary only if severe carditis is present
B the administration of prednisolone reduces the risk of permanent valvar disease
C chronic valvar damage is more likely to develop than after chorea
D permanent joint damage does not occur
E the development of pericarditis implies a very poor prognosis

445
In mitral stenosis
A there is no history of rheumatic fever or chorea in half the patients
B the rise in left atrial pressure on exercise is less than expected in patients with a raised pulmonary arteriolar resistance
C symptoms may be alleviated by pregnancy
D haemoptysis is a recognised complication
E systemic embolism does not occur unless atrial fibrillation is present

446
Recognised features of pure mitral stenosis include
A a prominent 'a' wave in the jugular venous pulse
B a loud pulmonary second sound
C a heaving apical impulse
D a tall P wave in the electrocardiogram
E enlargement of the left atrium to both left and right in the chest X-ray

447
Mitral valvotomy
A carries a prohibitive risk during pregnancy
B may result in mitral regurgitation
C may require cardiopulmonary bypass
D is more likely to be successful if the valve is uncalcified
E should precede an attempt at medical treatment of associated heart failure

448
Recognised causes of the sudden development of mitral regurgitation include
A infective endocarditis
B myxomatous degeneration of the valve
C myocardial infarction
D rheumatic fever
E rupture of the chordae tendineae

449
Pure aortic stenosis
A is characterised by a progressive fall in cardiac output as the stenosis increases in severity
B may result from an accelerated ageing process in a congenital bicuspid valve
C is a recognised cause of syncope
D is a recognised cause of a large 'a' wave in the jugular venous pulse
E should not be treated surgically until the patient complains of dyspnoea

450
In aortic regurgitation
A angina does not occur unless there is coexistent coronary atheroma
B there is a systolic pressure gradient across the aortic valve
C a basal diastolic thrill is typically present
D the murmur is best heard with the patient recumbent and rolled towards the left
E the left ventricular stroke output may be increased up to three-fold

451
Tricuspid stenosis
A is more commonly of congenital than of rheumatic origin
B produces a diastolic murmur similar to that of aortic regurgitation
C is unlikely to be present in the absence of a peaked P wave in the electrocardiogram
D when rheumatic in origin, usually implies that severe pancarditis has been present
E is a recognised cause of ascites

452
Tricuspid regurgitation
A may result from myocardial ischaemia
B usually requires valve replacement
C causes a large 'a' wave in the jugular venous pulse
D may cause systolic expansion of the liver
E is a recognised feature of chronic cor pulmonale

453
Characteristic features of isolated pulmonary stenosis include
A central cyanosis
B a systolic murmur and thrill to the left of the upper sternum
C an ejection sound
D an increased right ventricular thrust
E a loud pulmonary second sound

454
In infective endocarditis
A stenosed valves are more commonly àffected than regurgitant lesions
B glomerulonephritis is probably due to an immune-complex reaction
C blood for culture should be taken only during a rise in the patient's temperature
D the common portal of entry of *Streptococcus viridans* is infected paranasal sinuses
E normal valves are not affected

455
Features which suggest a diagnosis of infective endocarditis in a patient with a valve lesion include
A unusual tiredness
B night sweats
C a palpable spleen
D venous thrombosis in the legs
E hypochromic microcytic anaemia

456
In the treatment of infective endocarditis
A infection with *Streptococcus viridans* is best treated with penicillin and probenecid
B co-trimoxazole is the first choice antibiotic if no organism is isolated
C infection with *Streptococcus faecalis* is best treated with gentamicin in addition to penicillin and probenecid
D infection with *Coxiella burnetti* usually responds to penicillin
E infection on a prosthetic valve must be eradicated before replacing the valve

457
The left coronary artery
A supplies the whole of the interventricular septum
B supplies the SA node
C is unlikely to be normal if angina is present
D divides into anterior descending and circumflex branches
E supplies the inferior part of the left ventricle

458
Angina pectoris is a recognised feature of
A aortic stenosis
B polyarteritis
C paroxysmal tachycardia
D Mönckeberg's sclerosis
E anaemia

459
In a patient with central chest pain
A the absence of abnormal physical signs is very much against a diagnosis of angina
B ST depression of 2mm in an electrocardiogram recorded after exercise is much in favour of ischaemic heart disease
C provocation of the pain by exercise is very strong evidence of ischaemic heart disease
D of burning quality, oesophagitis is the probable diagnosis
E the gestures with which he indicates the site of the pain may be of diagnostic significance

460
In the treatment of angina pectoris
A regular exercise should be encouraged to promote the development of a collateral circulation
B over 20 per cent of patients are improved by placebos
C glyceryl trinitrate should be taken only when the pain is present
D propranolol should be withdrawn immediately if the patient becomes breathless
E aorto-coronary bypass surgery is contra-indicated by multiple coronary arterial obstructions

461
Symptoms compatible with a diagnosis of myocardial infarction include
A pain and numbness in a pale cold foot
B syncope
C tiredness
D dyspnoea
E vomiting

462
Within six hours of the onset of pain due to myocardial infarction typical corroborative findings include
A raised jugular venous pressure
B pericardial friction
C a fourth heart sound
D elevation of the ST segment in the electrocardiogram
E raised serum lactic dehydrogenase activity

463
In patients who have had a myocardial infarction
A an initial rise in blood pressure is commoner than a fall
B there is a 60 per cent mortality rate within a few minutes
C rupture of a mitral papillary muscle is indicated by the sudden development of a loud apical diastolic murmur
D pulmonary embolism is the commonest clinical manifestation of detached endocardial thrombus
E a syndrome of fever, pericarditis and pleurisy is a recognised late complication

464
In the treatment of myocardial infarction
A cyclizine should be given with opiates to prevent vomiting
B frequent ventricular extrasystoles should be treated unless they are of the 'R on T' variety
C sinus bradycardia may require treatment with atropine
D lignocaine is the drug of choice for the treatment of ventricular tachycardia
E atrial arrhythmias are best treated with mexiletine

465
Following a myocardial infarction
A endocardial thrombosis can be prevented by treatment with warfarin
B the patient should be kept in bed for at least two weeks
C much the commonest cause of permanent inability to work is severe angina
D patients who have required defibrillation for ventricular fibrillation are less likely to survive one year than those who have not
E one in four of those patients who leave hospital survive for 20 years

466
With regard to arterial blood pressure,
A the highest level is at least twice the lowest during 24 hours
B a single high casual recording has no correlation with life expectancy
C in middle age the systolic pressure is as good a prognostic indicator as the diastolic
D the majority of people with hypertension are symptomless
E essential hypertension is especially frequent in Japanese

467
The following statements about hypertension are correct:
A In the majority of patients renal disease is the cause
B In most cases there is another affected member of the family
C Plasma renin activity is raised in severe essential hypertension
D Low plasma renin activity and low serum potassium concentration together suggest an excess of circulating aldosterone
E Oral contraceptives may have an aetiological role

468
In a patient with hypertension the following physical signs may provide a clue to its cause:
A a loud aortic second sound
B a fourth heart sound
C basal crepitations
D a systolic bruit in the abdomen
E palpable kidneys

469
In the investigation of a patient with hypertension
A the electrocardiogram provides more reliable evidence of left ventricular hypertrophy than the chest X-ray
B unilateral renal disease is more readily demonstrated by excretion urography than by radio-isotope studies
C evidence of coarctation of the aorta may be found in the chest X-ray
D estimation of the plasma urate may provide evidence of the cause
E tall R waves in leads V1 and V2 of the electrocardiogram would be expected

470
The following drugs have anti-renin activity:
A propranolol
B clonidine
C methyldopa
D debrisoquine
E bendrofluazide

471
When used in the treatment of hypertension, propranolol
A may cause impotence
B should not be given with a diuretic
C is particularly valuable if angina pectoris coexists
D should not be given in a daily dosage of more than 100mg
E may cause bronchospasm

472
An appropriate line of treatment of
A hypertensive encephalopathy is intravenous diazoxide
B an asymptomatic 30 years old man with a diastolic pressure of 120mm Hg is rest and sedation
C a 70 year old woman with a diastolic pressure of 110mmHg is bethanidine
D mild hypertension is a thiazide diuretic with potassium supplements
E hypertension with co-existent renal failure is frusemide

473
Recognised causes of pulmonary arterial hypertension include
A mitral stenosis
B pulmonary regurgitation
C repetitive pulmonary thromboembolism
D chronic hypoxaemia
E persistent ductus arteriosus

474
Recognised features of primary pulmonary hypertension include
A a greater prevalence in men than women
B syncope on exertion
C tall R waves in lead V1 of the electrocardiogram
D a tendency to occur in families
E spontaneous remission within a few years in most cases

475
Characteristic features of massive pulmonary embolism include
A ischaemic cardiac pain
B haemoptysis
C pulmonary vascular congestion in the chest X-ray
D cyanosis
E pleural effusion

476
Heparin
A should be given intravenously in patients with venous thrombosis in the legs
B should be avoided if pulmonary embolism has caused severe hypotension
C can be given subcutaneously to prevent post-operative venous thrombosis
D is more likely to cause haemorrhage if the patient is also on salicylates
E is a thrombolytic drug

477
Cardiomyopathy
A is usually associated with acute pericarditis
B can simulate aortic stenosis
C of the congestive type can be treated with betareceptor blocking drugs
D of the hypertrophic type is usually due to alcoholism
E is commonly complicated by arrhythmias

478
Acute pericarditis
A is most often due to rheumatic fever in Britain
B causes pain which is indistinguishable from that of myocardial infarction
C produces friction which is best heard over the apical impulse
D is associated with ST elevation with upward concavity in the electrocardiogram
E is usually painless when due to uraemia

479
A pericardial effusion
A of 2 litres could well cause pulsus paradoxus
B of 300 ml is difficult to detect clinically
C which is purulent is usually very large
D could well be malignant if it is haemorrhagic
E should be aspirated unless it is due to tuberculosis

480
Characteristic features of chronic constrictive pericarditis include
A severe dyspnoea
B tachycardia
C a normal sized heart associated with a very high venous pressure
D a third heart sound
E pericardial calcification

481
Congenital heart disease
A occurs in about 1 per cent of live births
B is due, in most cases, to maternal rubella
C can be complicated by infective endocarditis
D with central cyanosis in the neonate is most commonly due to Fallot's tetralogy
E is unlikely to be associated with cyanosis in older children in the absence of pulmonary stenosis or pulmonary vascular disease

482
Recognised features of the following varieties of congenital heart disease include:
A Persistent ductus arteriosus—a murmur loudest in mid systole
B Coarctation of the aorta—notching of the ribs by the dilated internal mammary artery visible on X-ray
C Atrial septal defect—cyanosis in early infancy
D Ventricular septal defect—left ventricular failure
E Fallot's tetralogy—squatting after exercise.

483
Radiological evidence of enlargement of the pulmonary artery is a recognised feature of
A mitral stenosis
B persistent ductus arteriosus
C atrial septal defect
D Fallot's tetralogy
E pulmonary valve stenosis

484
The following statements regarding cardiac surgery are correct:
A Recurrence of mitral stenosis is to be expected within 10 years even after a successful valvotomy.
B After infarction of a mitral papillary muscle, insertion of a valve prosthesis should not be deferred for longer than a week
C Haemolysis is a recognised complication of aortic valve prosthesis
D The heart cannot be stopped for more than an hour during bypass surgery.
E Homograft valves are less likely than prostheses to cause thromboembolism

485
Elective general surgery
A should be deferred until after mitral valvotomy
B should not be performed if the patient is on antihypertensive therapy
C should rarely be performed within three months of a myocardial infarction
D should, if possible, precede replacement of the mitral valve with a prosthesis
E is most safely performed in patients with heart disease if barbiturate induction of anaesthesia is used

486
In a pregnant woman
A mitral stenosis is an indication for termination
B with heart disease an uncomplicated delivery can be expected if she is symptom-free at 24 weeks
C who is cyanosed on account of a ventricular septal defect, early termination is indicated
D angina is the commonest manifestation of heart disease
E in whom a persistent ductus was ligated in childhood no problems are likely to arise

487
In long-standing occlusive arterial disease of the lower limbs
A loss of hair on the affected limb is a recognised feature
B a bruit may be audible over an area of narrowing
C pain at night is relieved by elevating the foot of the bed
D Mönckeberg's sclerosis is the most likely cause in the elderly
E regular exercise should be advised

488
An aneurysm
A of the ascending aorta is usually due to tertiary syphilis
B of the abdominal aorta is usually due to atherosclerosis
C in Marfan's syndrome is usually due to dissection
D of the ascending aorta may cause hoarseness of the voice
E of the arch of the aorta may erode ribs

489
Syphilitic aortitis
A is a recognised cause of myocardial ischaemia
B can lead to aortic stenosis
C is associated with calcification of the ascending aorta
D is characterised histologically by replacement of elastic tissue by fibrous tissue
E should be treated with benzylpenicillin and probenecid for 4-6 weeks

490
The following are more common in females than in males:
A thromboangiitis obliterans
B Takayashu's syndrome
C primary Raynaud's disease
D atrial septal defect
E coarctation of the aorta

491
Characteristic features of cranial arteritis include
A blindness
B diminished or absent arterial pulsation in the arms, head and neck
C pain and stiffness in the shoulders
D a rapid response to treatment with prednisolone
E a tendency to affect persons in the second and third decades of life predominantly

492
Recognised features of polyarteritis include
A eosinophilia
B asthma
C haematuria
D hypertension
E tender thickened peripheral arteries

493
Raynaud's phenomenon
A is a recognised cause of cryoglobulinaemia
B affects the fingers more than the toes
C responds consistently to vasodilator drugs
D does not cause irreversible ischaemic damage
E may be improved by sympathectomy especially if the toes are predominantly affected

494
Recognised causes of venous thrombosis in the legs include
A treatment with phenylbutazone
B malignant disease
C wearing elastic stockings
D the use of the contraceptive pill
E polycythaemia

495
A patient in the post-operative period
A is unlikely to have a deep venous thrombosis if there has been no pyrexia
B should be encouraged to exercise his legs regularly
C whose left leg is pinker and warmer than the right may well have a left deep venous thrombosis
D who develops a deep venous thrombosis should be nursed with the head of the bed raised for 48 hours
E should be given protamine sulphate if bleeding occurs while he is on warfarin

CHAPTER SEVEN

496
In normal man
A the trachea bifurcates at the level of the suprasternal notch
B the left main bronchus is more vertical than the right
C the lingular branch of the left upper lobe bronchus corresponds to the middle lobe bronchus on the right
D the middle lobe bronchus divides into medial and lateral branches
E cilia are present in the bronchial epithelium down as far as the segmental divisions

497
The following statements are correct:
A The left lung is divided into upper and lower lobes by the oblique fissure
B The transverse fissure runs horizontally from the junction of the 6th costal cartilage with the sternum to join the oblique fissure at the tip of the scapula
C The left upper lobe is largely in front of the lower lobe
D The middle lobe is situated behind the right upper lobe
E The parietal pleura is continuous with the visceral pleura at the pulmonary hilum

498
At rest in an adult the normal
A pulmonary blood flow is about 5l/min
B pulmonary ventilation is about 6l/min
C alveolar ventilation is about 3l/min (83-98mmHg)
D range of arterial PCO_2 is 4.8-6.0kPa (36-45mmHg)
E alveolar ventilation is about 3l/min

499
The 'elastic' work of breathing is increased in patients with
A pulmonary oedema
B bronchial asthma
C pulmonary fibrosis
D ankylosing spondylitis
E partial obstruction of a major bronchus by carcinoma

500
The following statements are correct:
A Breathing normally accounts for a small fraction of metabolic oxygen uptake
B Alveolar ventilation can be calculated from the product of tidal volume and respiratory rate
C Alveolar underventilation causes hypocapnia
D Alveolar underventilation causes hypoxaemia
E The changes in blood gas pressures produced by alveolar underventilation can be corrected by breathing oxygen

501
Alveolar underventilation typically occurs in
A salicylate overdosage
B severe chronic bronchitis
C interstitial lung disease
D pulmonary embolism
E kyphoscoliosis

502
In connection with the control of breathing
A pyrexia decreases the sensitivity of the respiratory centre
B a rise in the arterial PCO_2 stimulates both peripheral and central chemoreceptors
C chemoreceptor cells in the carotid body are sensitive to alterations in the arterial oxygen tension
D an increase in the hydrogen-ion activity of arterial blood causes chemoreceptors in the aortic body to stimulate respiration
E in severe chronic bronchitis the sensitivity of the respiratory centre to an increased arterial PCO_2 is enhanced

503
Pulmonary alveoli with
A a very high ventilation: perfusion $(\dot{V}A/\dot{Q})$ ratio contribute to the physiological dead space
B a very low $\dot{V}A/\dot{Q}$ ratio are associated with arterial hypoxaemia
C a low $\dot{V}A/\dot{Q}$ ratio are found in the segments distal to a pulmonary embolus
D a high $\dot{V}A/\dot{Q}$ ratio are found more in the lower lobes than the upper lobes of the lungs in the erect position
E a low $\dot{V}A/\dot{Q}$ ratio contain gas with a low PO_2 which cannot be corrected by the administration of oxygen.

504
The gas transfer factor
A is a precise measure of the rate at which oxygen and carbon dioxide diffuse across the alveolar membrane
B is determined by relating the uptake of CO by the blood to the alveolar CO pressure when a weak mixture of this gas is breathed
C is reduced in emphysema
D is uninfluenced by changes in the $\dot{V}A/\dot{Q}$ ratio
E is above normal in interstitial lung disease

505
Characteristic features of severe hypercapnia (arterial PCO_2 more than 11kPa or 80mmHg) include
A headache
B muscle twitching
C cold clammy skin
D drowsiness
E papilloedema

506
Recognised causes of Type 1 respiratory failure (arterial PCO_2 normal or low) include
A chronic bronchitis
B bronchial asthma
C pulmonary oedema
D fibrosing alveolitis
E severe kyphoscoliosis

507
Finger clubbing is a recognised feature of
A lung cancer
B bronchiectasis
C emphysema
D primary pulmonary tuberculosis
E cirrhosis of the liver

508
Breath sounds are diminished or absent over a
A pneumothorax
B pleural effusion
C consolidated lobe
D collapsed lobe to which the bronchus is occluded
E bronchiectatic lobe

509
The following statements are correct:
A Tomography is of particular value in defining cavitated lesions of the lungs
B A postero-anterior chest radiograph will accurately define the size and shape of the heart
C A false positive tuberculin test occurs in patients with sarcoidosis
D The range of vision with a fibreoptic bronchoscope is greater than that with the rigid type
E Lung biopsy can be performed only by formal thoracotomy

510
The ratio of FEV$_1$ to FVC
A is a useful way of assessing the severity of a restrictive ventilatory defect
B is increased in chronic bronchitis
C is decreased in ankylosing spondylitis
D can be increased by the inhalation of salbutamol in asthma
E is probably less than 50 per cent if forced expiratory time is more than six seconds

511
Oxygen
A is present in air at a concentration of 21 per cent
B in high concentration overcomes the hypoxaemia consequent upon a high alveolar PCO_2
C in inspired tracheal air is at a pressure of about 20kPa (150mmHg)
D may safely be given to adults in 100 per cent concentration indefinitely
E may damage the eyes when given in high concentration to premature infants

512
The following statements are correct:
A The MC mask will deliver 60 per cent oxygen at a flow rate of 4-6 1/min
B The convenience of nasal catheters is offset because of the need to humidify the inspired oxygen
C The Ventimask produces oxygen enrichment of the inspired air without rebreathing of expired carbon dioxide
D Oxygen tents are of particular value in the treatment of adults because of the consistent oxygen concentration delivered
E Oxygen should be given intermittently to confused or restless patients

513
In the treatment of a patient with acute ventilatory failure
A a tracheostomy should be performed if mechanical ventilation is needed for more than 12 hours
B a cannula can be left in the radial or brachial artery for obtaining repeated blood samples
C up to 60 per cent oxygen can be given during mechanical ventilation
D mechanical ventilation can be discontinued as soon as the disturbances in PaO_2, $PaCO_2$ and pH have been corrected
E diazepam is the drug of choice if sedation is required

514
In the treatment of a chronic bronchitic with persistent hypoxaemia and hypercapnia

A doxapram by inhalation has a worthwhile bronchodilator effect

B oral dichlorphenamide should be prescribed

C a worthwhile increase in exercise tolerance can result from the use of portable oxygen equipment

D an unproductive cough which disturbs his sleep should be suppressed with pholcodine or methadone linctus

E hot drinks may help him bring up tenacious sputum

515
The following statements are correct:

A A throat swab gives the best yield in the identification of a virus infecting the respiratory tract

B A four-fold rise in titre of antibody in paired sera suggests a recent infection with the virus concerned

C Otitis media is a recognised complication of acute coryza

D Herpangina is a recognised manifestation of Coxsackie A viral infection

E Children with acute laryngotracheobronchitis should be given an antibiotic

516
The following organisms are paired with the disorder they are known to cause:

A Adenoviruses—acute laryngitis

B Echoviruses—pharyngoconjunctival fever

C Coxsackie viruses—laryngotracheobronchitis

D Influenza virus C—acute coryza

E *Coxiella burneti*—primary pneumonia

517
Pharyngoconjunctival fever

A can be distinguished from infectious mononucleosis by the absence of enlarged cervical lymph nodes

B is clinically indistinguishable from acute streptococcal sore throat

C should be treated with an antibiotic to prevent secondary bacterial infection

D is commonly due to an adenovirus

E can cause paroxysmal cough with dyspnoea and stridor

518
Influenza A viral infection

A is followed by life-long immunity

B may be complicated by sudden death due to a related cardiomyopathy

C is apt to be followed by bacterial pneumonia

D can be prevented in 70 per cent of individuals by specific vaccination

E is typically associated with a lymphocytosis

519
Characteristic features of acute tracheo-bronchitis include

A a loose productive cough initially

B retrosternal discomfort

C wheezy breathing

D a neutrophil leucocytosis

E bilateral rhonchi

520
Characteristic features of pneumococcal pneumonia include

A a peak frequency in the elderly

B homogeneous consolidation of one or more bronchopulmonary segments

C highest incidence in the early spring

D early onset of pleuritic pain

E a high incidence of associated herpes labialis

521
Recognised complications of pneumococcal pneumonia include

A empyema

B bronchial carcinoma

C peripheral circulatory failure

D pericarditis

E subphrenic abscess

522
The following statements are correct:
A Staphylococcal infection is a recognised complication of influenza
B Staphylococcal pneumonia usually responds to treatment with penicillin
C Klebsiella pneumonia typically causes massive consolidation and excavation of one or more lobes.
D Cold agglutinins are demonstrable in a high proportion of patients with *Mycoplasma pneumoniae* infections
E Chickenpox pneumonia is commoner in children than in adults

523
Pneumonia
A which is followed by miliary calcification was probably due to the measles virus
B due to *Chlamydia* is transmitted to humans by infected bird faeces
C in psittacosis is best treated with ampicillin
D due to the respiratory syncytial virus has a high mortality in the neonatal period
E due to *Coxiella burneti* may be complicated by endocarditis

524
Pneumonia is more likely to be due to a virus or small bacterium than to the pneumococcus if
A physical signs in the chest are inconspicuous
B respiratory symptoms precede fever and toxaemia
C the spleen is palpable
D the white blood count is normal
E a pleural effusion develops

525
The following statements about aspiration pneumonias are correct:
A Bronchiectasis is a recognised sequela of bronchopneumonia
B Acute lobular pneumonia is a recognised complication of chronic bronchitis
C Benign aspiration pneumonia complicating coryza typically causes bilateral symmetrical radiographic opacities
D Hypostatic pneumonia in elderly patients characteristically has an acute onset
E Pulmonary abscess may result from bacterial infection of a collapsed lobe

526
Pulmonary abscess
A following an operation on the nose is characteristically situated in the basal segments of the lower lobes
B typically causes a high remittent pyrexia
C may result from infection of a pulmonary infarct
D may result from obstruction of a bronchus by carcinoma
E may be simulated by a cavitated malignant tumour

527
The following diseases are paired with their specific antimicrobial therapy:
A Pneumococcal pneumonia— co-trimoxazole
B Klebsiella pneumonia—sodium fusidate
C Mycoplasma pneumonia—tetracycline
D Staphylococcal pneumonia—ampicillin
E *Coxiella burneti* infection—cephalexin

528
In Western Europe tuberculosis
A develops more often in those under the age of 40 than in older age groups
B is more common in diabetics than in the general population
C can be expected to advance rapidly in pregnancy even in patients who are being correctly treated
D is commoner in males than females
E is due to the bovine bacillus as often as it is to the human

529
Primary tuberculous infection
A typically causes a protracted febrile illness
B is almost always associated with caseation in the regional lymph nodes
C typically causes unilateral hilar lymph node enlargement
D may be complicated by acute miliary spread
E can be excluded by a negative tuberculin test

530
Miliary tuberculosis
A in young adults characteristically causes a fever with drenching night sweats
B may be diagnosed by liver biopsy
C can be confirmed by the presence of iridocyclitis on ophthalmoscopy
D is characteristically associated with a polymorph leucocytosis
E in the 'cryptic' form may present with symptoms of anaemia only

531
In post-primary pulmonary tuberculosis
A the lesions are most frequently found in the lower lobes
B spontaneous pneumothorax may mark the onset of the disease
C a lesion detected radiologically is probably inactive if the patient has no symptoms
D haemoptysis occurs only in the later stages
E crepitations heard only after coughing are a recognised feature

532
Recognised complications of pulmonary tuberculosis include
A bronchiectasis
B ischiorectal abscess
C sarcoidosis
D ventilatory failure
E mycetoma

533
The following statements relating to the treatment of pulmonary tuberculosis are correct:
A Persistence of a positive sputum culture after six months treatment can only be due to drug resistance
B Intermittent twice weekly drug regimens are of particular value in unco-operative patients
C Drugs should always be prescribed in combination
D Economic necessity justifies the use of isoniazid and thiacetazone in combination in developing countries
E Isoniazid should not be given with either rifampicin or ethambutol

534
The following anti-tuberculous drugs are recognised causes of the side-effects listed with them:
A streptomycin—renal failure
B PAS—polyneuropathy
C isoniazid—hypothyroidism
D rifampicin—hepatitis
E thiacetazone—leucopenia

535
The following statements concerning the treatment of tuberculosis are correct:
A The administration of rifampicin can cause severe bleeding in patients on anticoagulants
B For miliary tuberculosis twelve months treatment is sufficient
C Genito-urinary tuberculosis requires 18 months treatment even if rifampicin is given throughout
D Corticosteroids should be used only when there is ocular involvement
E Capreomycin is useful in the case of infections resistant to other drugs

536
In the prevention of tuberculosis chemoprophylaxis with isoniazid is indicated in
A insulin-dependent diabetics
B patients on immunosuppressive drugs
C tuberculin-positive children under three years of age
D individuals living in lodging houses
E individuals who have recently become tuberculin-positive

537
Recognised consequences of pulmonary infection with *Aspergillus fumigatus* include
A recurrent haemoptyses
B allergic alveolitis
C bronchial asthma
D pulmonary necrosis
E cyst and bulla formation in the lung

538
The following statements about hypersensitivity reactions in the respiratory tract are correct:
A The Type I response is manifest clinically as allergic alveolitis
B Bronchial asthma is due to an immediate reaction
C The Type III response is mediated by precipitating antibody (IgG)
D The Type IV response is cell-mediated and usually associated with delayed hypersensitivity
E Ingested antigens usually produce late hypersensitivity reactions

539
Allergic rhinitis is
A due to a Type II reaction
B commonest in Britain between May and July
C characterised by a purulent nasal discharge
D liable to subside spontaneously
E responsive to prophylactic treatment with sodium cromoglycate

540
Bronchial asthma
A in childhood is characteristically caused by a single specific allergen
B of late onset typically arises in atopic individuals
C in atopic individuals is typically due to inhaled allergens
D is more likely to be due to the ingestion of aspirin if it starts in middle age
E may be precipitated in predisposed individuals by strenuous exertion

541
The following statements about asthma are correct:
A Serial estimations of peak expiratory flow rate are of little value in monitoring response to treatment
B An eosinophilia is found only in status asthmaticus
C In chronic asthma the cough is typically unproductive
D During a paroxysm the chest is held in full inspiration
E Severe asthma starting in childhood usually causes a 'pigeon chest' deformity

542
In an acute asthmatic attack
A the patient should be nursed flat
B oxygen therapy is contra-indicated
C beta-adrenergic blocking agents are useful
D subcutaneous adrenaline is the initial treatment of choice
E oral prednisolone should be withheld while intravenous hydrocortisone is being administered

543
The following statements are correct:
A Intermittent positive pressure ventilation may be life-saving in status asthmaticus
B Dehydration is a common accompaniment of status asthmaticus
C Diazepam is a safe sedative in asthmatic patients on intermittent positive pressure ventilation
D The prophylactic administration of antihistamine drugs is effective in intrinsic asthma
E Hyposensitisation is of value in atopic asthmatics sensitive to house dust

544
Pulmonary eosinophilia is
A typically associated with blood eosinophilia
B a recognised association of ascariasis
C invariably associated with asthma
D a recognised sequel to sulphonamide administration
E characteristically associated with the presence of LE cells in the blood

545
Asthmatic pulmonary eosinophilia
A is due to allergic bronchopulmonary aspergillosis in over 50 per cent of cases
B can be effectively treated with diethylcarbamazine
C is due to a Type II allergic reaction
D is a recognised cause of bronchiectasis
E has many features in common with polyarteritis

546
The following statements are correct:
A Hoarseness is a feature of glossopharyngeal palsy
B A 'bovine' cough is characteristic of hysterical laryngeal paralysis
C Stridor is a typical feature of bilateral organic laryngeal paralysis
D A paralysed vocal cord lies in a fully abducted position
E Laryngeal obstruction may arise as a complication of rheumatoid arthritis

547
Characteristic features of chronic bronchitis include
A a lifelong history of recurrent acute bronchitis
B oversecretion of mucus
C a normal FEV_1/FVC ratio
D decreased residual volume
E a life expectancy of 10 years from the onset of symptoms at most

548
In chronic bronchitis
A antibiotic treatment of an acute exacerbation should rarely be started until bacteriological examination of the sputum has been carried out
B continuous antibiotic therapy should be given throughout the winter
C an unproductive cough may require suppression with pholcodine
D *Staph. pyogenes* is commoner than *Strept. pneumoniae* as a cause of infection
E the PaO_2 falls before the $PaCO_2$ rises

549
In emphysema
A without chronic bronchitis airways obstruction is not present
B with chronic bronchitis the distribution is usually centrilobular
C dyspnoea is typically more prominent than in chronic bronchitis
D cyanosis is an early manifestation
E in young adults α_1-antitrypsin deficiency is a recognised association

550
Typical findings in an emphysematous patient during inspiration include
A tracheal descent
B excavation of the suprasternal fossa
C jugular venous filling
D contraction of the scalene muscles
E indrawing of the costal margins

551
Typical findings in the chest radiograph in emphysema include
A prominent peripheral vascular markings
B 'inflammatory shadowing'
C a low flat diaphragm
D prominent pulmonary arteries at the hila
E bullae

552
Recognised features of bronchiectasis include
A night sweats
B episodes of pleurisy
C empyema
D haemoptysis
E crepitations audible over affected segments

553
In the treatment of bronchiectasis
A postural drainage is only worthwhile if it can be continued for at least an hour at a time
B surgical treatment must be preceded by bronchography
C emphysema is a contra-indication to surgery
D failure of medical treatment is a clear indication for surgery
E the most successful surgical results are in children and young adults

554
The following statements are correct:
A Mediastinal displacement towards the affected side is a typical feature of main bronchus obstruction
B A partially obstructed main bronchus may lead to displacement of the mediastinum away from the affected side on inspiration
C Bacterial infection distal to a partially obstructed bronchus is unusual unless there is associated pulmonary collapse
D Enlarged lymph nodes may mimic intra-luminal bronchial obstruction
E Obstructive emphysema is more likely to result from bronchial carcinoma than adenoma

555
Bronchial carcinoma
A accounts for 10 per cent of all male deaths from cancer
B is as common in women as men after the age of 50 years
C is ten times more common among coal miners than in the general population
D is thirty times more common as a cause of death in heavy smokers than in non-smokers
E characteristically presents with massive haemoptysis

556
The following statements are correct:
A Horner's syndrome is a recognised complication of an apical bronchial carcinoma
B Haematuria may be the presenting feature of a bronchial carcinoma
C 'Oat cell' carcinomas may act as an ectopic source of antidiuretic hormone
D The outlook is more favourable when a bronchial tumour is of 'oat cell' type
E A paralysed hemidiaphragm moves down when the patient sniffs

557
Bronchial carcinoma
A is usually so far distal that a positive bronchoscopic diagnosis can be made in no more than 20 per cent of cases
B can be excluded as the cause of haemoptysis if the chest radiograph is normal
C causes death in less than a year from diagnosis if resection is impossible
D has a five-year survival rate of 60 per cent after resection
E can be confidently treated by resection in about 50 per cent of patients

558
Recognised features of fibrosing alveolitis include
A widespread wheezing
B carbon dioxide retention
C finger clubbing
D a positive test for rheumatoid factor
E recurrent haemoptyses

559
Sarcoidosis
A is characterised by cavitated pulmonary lesions
B is typically associated with a strongly positive Mantoux reaction
C in its subacute form resolves spontaneously in most cases within two years
D may cause hypercalcaemia
E typically presents with erythema marginatum

560
Typical features of subacute sarcoidosis include
A bilateral parotid swelling
B cranial nerve palsies
C polyarthralgia
D iritis
E interstitial pulmonary fibrosis

561
The following occupations are associated with the diseases with which they are paired:
A farming—extrinsic allergic alveolitis
B the cane sugar industry—byssinosis
C the plastic and rubber industries—bronchial asthma
D tin mining—siderosis
E metal grinding—silicosis

562

The following statements are correct:

A Silicosis results from prolonged inhalation of coal dust

B Long exposure to dust containing iron or tin causes extensive pulmonary fibrosis

C Antinuclear factor (ANF) is present in the serum in about 15 per cent of patients with coal workers' pneumoconiosis

D Progressive massive fibrosis may cavitate

E 'Egg shell' calcification in the hilar lymph nodes is a characteristic feature of silicosis

563

The following statements about asbestosis are correct:

A The radiological abnormalities are most marked in the upper zones

B Peritoneal mesothelioma may follow trivial exposure to blue asbestos

C Blood-stained pleural effusion is a recognised complication

D Lung biopsy may be required to confirm the diagnosis

E The dust particles are so small that protective respirators are ineffective

564

In a patient with a pleural effusion

A breathlessness is unlikely to occur unless an effusion develops on the other side also

B the diagnosis can usually be made on clinical grounds alone

C percutaneous biopsy is rarely justifiable

D a tuberculous aetiology can be excluded if there is no radiologically apparent pulmonary disease

E and a history of recent upper respiratory infection, the finding of many lymphocytes in the fluid would suggest that the effusion is 'post-pneumonic'

565

Empyema thoracis

A typically involves the whole hemithorax

B complicated by a bronchopleural fistula is characterised by a horizontal 'fluid level' in the chest radiograph

C most commonly follows bacterial pneumonia

D may complicate a haemothorax

E is a recognised complication of subphrenic abscess

566

Spontaneous pneumothorax

A is a recognised complication of tuberculosis

B typically results from rupture of a subpleural bulla

C may complicate staphylococcal lung abscess

D may not produce any abnormal physical signs

E may not require any active treatment

567

The following statements are correct:

A Pectus carinatum is a recognised sequel to childhood tuberculosis

B Pectus excavatum results from chronic airways obstruction

C Severe thoracic kyphoscoliosis causes a rise in the $\dot{V}_A/\dot{Q}$ ratio

D Ventilatory failure is a recognised sequel to ankylosing spondylitis

E Pectus excavatum should be corrected in early childhood to ensure normal ventilatory function

CHAPTER EIGHT

568
The following statements regarding the control and co-ordination of the alimentary tract are correct:
A Sympathetic nerve fibres run in the splanchnic nerves
B The parasympathetic system is inhibitory
C The nervous system exerts an effect on the secretion of hormones by the mucosa
D The hormone gastrin is released initially in response to intake of food
E Exocrine pancreatic secretion is controlled both by nervous and hormonal factors

569
The following statements regarding gastrointestinal motility are correct:
A The upper oesophageal sphincter is closed except during swallowing
B The lower oesophageal sphincter is controlled solely by nervous mechanisms
C The normal tonic contraction of the stomach is increased when food enters it
D Gastric emptying is controlled by means of local reflexes
E In normal man approximately half of a semisolid meal has left the stomach within 15 minutes of ingestion

570
In the alimentary tract,
A the frequency of the 'slow wave' is greater in the ileum than in the duodenum
B the myenteric plexus and the enteric hormones determine the local response to the 'slow wave'
C propulsion of colonic contents is facilitated by segmentation
D colonic motor activity is inhibited after eating
E diarrhoea is associated with increased motor activity of the colon

571
The following statements concerning alimentary secretion are correct:
A Gastrin secretion is inhibited by a rise in intragastric pH
B Gastric secretion is stimulated by secretin and cholecystokinin—pancreozymin
C Secretin stimulates bicarbonate secretion by the acinar cells of the pancreas
D Cholecystokinin—pancreozymin causes contraction of the gall bladder
E The enteric hormones inhibit secretion of succus entericus

572
In the normal alimentary tract
A fat soluble vitamins are transported from the absorptive cell by the lymphatic system
B hexoses are transported from the absorptive cell by the portal venous system
C the epithelial surface of the small intestine is replaced every week
D phenylbutazone increases the rate of cell turnover in the stomach
E secretory IgA has a role in protecting mucosal surfaces from bacterial invasion

573
Vomiting
A in children is a recognised feature of infective illnesses
B without preceding nausea is a recognised feature of intracranial disease
C which is persistent and associated with weight loss is almost certainly due to malignant disease
D in the morning is typical of gastric outlet obstruction
E which relieves pain is a recognised feature of peptic ulcer

574
In normal Western man
A a plain X-ray of the abdomen shows that gas predominates in the small intestine
B fewer than 10 per cent of individuals have less than one bowel motion per day
C approximately 5 per cent of individuals have more than three bowel movements daily
D a gain in weight is incompatible with a diagnosis of peptic ulcer
E a high residue diet increases the incidence of constipation

575
Endoscopy
A is contra-indicated when barium swallow suggests an oesophageal tumour
B is of little diagnostic value in patients suffering from radiologically negative epigastric pain
C is of particular value in the assessment of patients with upper alimentary symptoms after gastric surgery
D should be avoided in fulminating ulcerative colitis
E using the sigmoidoscope demands careful bowel preparation over several days

576
The following statements regarding barium studies are correct:
A The addition of gas enhances the examination of the mucosal surface
B Radiological examination of the abdomen in women of child-bearing age should be confined to the 10 days immediately following the onset of the last menstrual period
C An inert area observed during observation of the motility of the stomach suggests infiltrative disease
D Clumping and flocculation of barium in the small intestine is a recognised feature of malabsorption
E In patients with ischaemic heart disease a barium enema may induce an arrhythmia

577
In the investigation of the alimentary tract
A colonic cytology is a valuable technique in the diagnosis of carcinoma of the colon
B small intestinal biopsy should always be preceded by estimation of the prothrombin time and a platelet count
C a very high basal gastric acid output is a recognised feature of the Zollinger-Ellison syndrome
D achlorhydria is diagnosed when the pH of the gastric juice does not fall below 6 after pentagastrin stimulation
E the pentagastrin test is of value in assessing the completeness of vagotomy

578
The following statements regarding stomatitis and gingivitis are correct:
A Phenytoin is a recognised cause of gum hypertrophy
B In acute stomatitis atrophy of the papillae of the tongue is characteristic
C Vincent's angina is caused by an exogenous viral infection
D Oral thrush is a recognised complication of corticosteroid therapy
E Aphthous stomatitis is a manifestation of Coxsackie virus infection

579
In the treatment of diseases of the mouth
A metronidazole is the drug of choice in aphthous stomatitis
B thrush responds to the local application of tincture of benzoin
C tetracycline is the treatment of choice for non-specific stomatitis
D Vincent's angina characteristically responds to treatment with local hydrocortisone
E extensive dental surgery may be required following an episode of ulcerative stomatitis

580
Recognised causes of stomatitis include
A psoriasis
B pemphigus
C erythema multiforme
D exposure to mercury
E allergy to toothpaste

581
The following statements are correct:
A The presence of fur on the tongue is a recognised association of untreated peptic ulcer
B Tertiary syphilis affecting the tongue is characterised by exquisitely painful ulcers
C Pain is a characteristic early feature of leukoplakia
D Leukoplakia is a pre-malignant condition
E The pain of acute glossitis is characteristically relieved by hot liquids

582
Recognised causes of excessive salivary secretion include
A sarcoidosis
B trigeminal neuralgia
C administration of anticholinergic drugs
D Sjögren's syndrome
E administration of potassium iodide

583
Recognised causes of dysphagia include
A oesophageal candidiasis
B systemic sclerosis
C myasthenia gravis
D diphtheritic neuritis
E pharyngeal pouch

584
Recognised features of sideropenic dysphagia (Plummer-Vinson syndrome) include
A hyperchlorhydria
B splenomegaly
C glossitis
D an association with an hysterical personality
E finger clubbing

585
Symptoms due to reflux oesophagitis
A respond poorly to alkalis
B are typically aggravated by bending
C may mimic ischaemic cardiac pain
D may be differentiated from those of duodenal ulcer by the fact that nocturnal pain is exceptional in oesophagitis
E respond to treatment with cimetidine

586
The following statements are correct:
A Progressive dysphagia is a characteristic feature of traction diverticulum of the oesophagus
B Pharyngeal pouch may present with recurrent attacks of stridor
C Pharyngeal pouch characteristically presents in early adult life
D Recurrent pneumonia may complicate pharyngeal pouch
E Patients with a pharyngeal pouch should be advised to sleep in a semi-upright position

587
Achalasia of the cardia
A is due to spasm of the cardiac sphincter with hypertrophy of the muscle above
B is characteristically associated with acid regurgitation
C is a recognised cause of recurrent pneumonitis
D is associated with an increased liability to carcinoma of the oesophagus
E shows an X-ray appearance during barium swallow that can be mimicked by carcinoma

588
Carcinoma of the oesophagus
A is more common in men than in women
B is rare in Southern Africa
C in the Western Hemisphere most commonly involves the upper third
D is typically an adenocarcinoma
E produces dysphagia which is typically poorly localised by the patient

589
Characteristic features of carcinoma of the oesophagus include
A progressive dysphagia
B late invasion of surrounding structures
C a surgical cure rate of approximately 30 per cent
D a later age of onset than most other cancers
E acid regurgitation

590
The following factors have been shown to have a significant association with peptic ulcer:
A gastric hypersecretion
B pernicious anaemia
C bile reflux
D mental stress
E the use of an oral contraceptive preparation containing oestrogen and progestogen

591
Regarding peptic ulcer,
A the proportion of gastric to duodenal ulcer is higher in Scotland than in London
B in Britain ulcer mortality is highest in August and September
C active ulcers are virtually unknown during pregnancy
D benign gastric ulcers occur most commonly on the greater curvature
E the prevalence of duodenal ulcer in women compared with that in men has increased since the early years of this century

592
Chronic peptic ulcer
A may present with any of its complications with no previous history
B of the duodenum characteristically occurs within 1 cm of the pylorus
C pain is not referred to the back unless penetration posteriorly has occurred
D may present with nausea and anorexia
E of the duodenum occurs most commonly in patients of the upper socio-economic classes

593
The pain of peptic ulcer
A is typically described by the patient as 'stabbing'
B is characteristically periodic
C is relieved by antacids in approximately 50 per cent of cases
D of the duodenum characteristically occurs within one hour of eating
E of the duodenum is characteristically relieved by food

594
The following statements regarding peptic ulcer are correct:
A Relief of symptoms is closely correlated with ulcer healing
B The 'pointing sign', when associated with localised tenderness, is practically diagnostic of peptic ulcer
C The rate of healing can be accelerated by a bland ulcer diet
D There is good evidence that smoking retards the healing of gastric ulcer
E Hourly feeding of milk provokes less acid secretion in the stomach than does a diet of three main meals a day

595
Regarding the treatment of peptic ulcer
A non-absorbable antacids provide more rapid relief of pain than does sodium bicarbonate
B aluminium antacids lead to diarrhoea
C magnesium compounds are contra-indicated in patients with renal failure
D cimetidine is associated with a significant incidence of bone marrow suppression
E cimetidine is the treatment of choice for uncomplicated duodenal ulcer

596
The following statements are correct:
A Propantheline has been shown to accelerate the rate of healing of gastric ulcer
B Carbenoxolone has been proved to accelerate the rate of healing of duodenal ulcer
C Potassium depletion is a recognised unwanted effect of carbenoxolone therapy
D Carbenoxolone is contra-indicated in hypertensive patients
E Tranquillisers such as diazepam should be avoided in the treatment of patients with peptic ulcer

597
Indications for elective surgery in the treatment of peptic ulcer include
A gastric outlet obstruction
B recurrent ulcer following previous gastric surgery
C a gastric ulcer that has failed to heal after four weeks medical treatment
D persistent symptoms which, despite medical treatment, reduce the patient's capacity to work
E hour-glass stomach

598
Regarding elective surgery in peptic ulcer,
A proximal gastric vagotomy must be accompanied by a drainage procedure
B in patients with a low acid output, gastroenterostomy without vagotomy is a suitable procedure
C vagotomy carries a higher incidence of long-term complications than does partial gastrectomy
D following truncal vagotomy, vagal innervation of the small intestine is preserved
E constipation is a characteristic late complication of vagotomy

599
Gastroduodenal haemorrhage
A when due to peptic ulcer carries a mortality of approximately 20 per cent
B in Britain is more commonly due to oesophageal varices than to chronic gastric ulcer
C should be investigated by barium meal rather than by endoscopy in the first instance
D from acute ulceration is a recognised sequel to extensive burns
E can be caused by the ingestion of aspirin

600
Recognised features of acute gastroduodenal haemorrhage include
A passage of red blood per rectum
B restlessness and disorientation
C a falling haemoglobin level over several days in the absence of evidence of continued bleeding
D angina
E syncope preceding any other evidence of bleeding

601
In the management of a patient with a major gastroduodenal haemorrhage
A morphine is the sedative of choice
B a naso-gastric tube should be passed
C blood transfusion should be avoided unless the haemoglobin is less than 12 g/dl
D cimetidine has no place
E emergency surgery should be advised in most patients over 50 who bleed again after admission

602
The following statements regarding perforation of a peptic ulcer are correct:
A The complication is more commonly due to gastric than to duodenal ulcer
B About one quarter of all perforations occur in acute ulcers
C A period of temporary improvement in the patient's condition several hours after the onset is characteristic
D Shoulder tip pain is a recognised feature
E More than half the patients treated by a simple closure operation will subsequently require a further elective operation for recurrence of ulcer symptoms

603
Recognised features of gastric outlet obstruction include
A prompt relief of symptoms by vomiting
B acidosis
C tetany
D visible gastric peristalsis
E vomiting of bile when the obstruction is due to chronic duodenal ulceration

604
In the treatment of gastric outlet obstruction
A gastric aspiration should be carried out every 2 to 4 hours for at least 3 days
B intravenous fluids should be limited to 2 litres a day because of the risk of fluid overload
C potassium should be avoided in the infusion fluid
D if there is symptomatic improvement with medical treatment surgery will usually not be necessary
E parenteral vitamins should be given to all but the mildest cases

D

605
Characteristic features of the Zollinger-Ellison syndrome include
A diarrhoea
B an exaggerated increase in the acid secretory rate following pentagastrin
C jejunal ulceration
D a normal volume of fasting gastric juice of very low pH
E gastric mucosal atrophy

606
Recognised complications of surgery performed for duodenal ulcer include
A jejunal ulcer
B gastro-jejuno-colic fistula
C biliary gastritis
D constipation
E osteoporosis

607
The dumping syndrome
A is typically associated with intense drowsiness coupled with muscular weakness
B characteristically causes symptoms 1-2 hours after a meal
C is probably related to rapid gastric emptying
D is characteristically associated with peripheral vasoconstriction
E tends to become less troublesome with time

608
After an operation on the stomach
A about 50 per cent of patients feel distended and uncomfortable during and after a meal
B anaemia does not occur after vagotomy alone
C the incidence of iron deficiency anaemia reaches a peak 12 to 18 months after surgery
D post-operative diarrhoea may respond to a short course of tetracycline
E osteomalacia may not become clinically apparent until 15-20 years after partial gastrectomy

609
Acute gastritis
A is most commonly caused by the ingestion of irritant materials such as alcohol
B can usually be diagnosed from the thickened mucosal folds seen in the barium meal
C characteristically leads to permanent histological changes in the gastric mucosa
D is associated with increased acid output by the parietal cells
E may complicate septicaemia

610
Chronic gastritis
A of the atrophic variety is characterised by symptoms which mimic gastric ulcer
B is a characteristic finding in pernicious anaemia
C if severe, may be diagnosed by barium meal examination
D responds well to treatment with carbenoxolone
E is a recognised association of gastric carcinoma

611
Carcinoma of the stomach
A is commoner in the U.S.A. than in Japan
B complicates pernicious anaemia in less than 2 per cent of cases
C is a recognised long term hazard in patients with achlorhydria following gastric surgery
D may cause diarrhoea due to rapid gastric emptying
E presenting as an ulcer can be diagnosed with certainty only by gastroscopy and biopsy

612
Recognised features of carcinoma of the stomach include
A supraclavicular lymph node enlargement
B dysphagia
C spread to the duodenal mucosa with symptoms of duodenal ulcer
D an elevated E.S.R.
E presentation as an iron deficiency anaemia

613
The following statements regarding carcinoma of the stomach are correct:
A Exfoliative cytology has no place in the diagnosis
B Two thirds of patients coming to laparotomy have tumours capable of radical removal
C When pyloric obstruction is present surgery is to be recommended even if there are secondary deposits
D The prognosis over the last 40 years has shown significant improvement as a result of new surgical techniques
E When complicated by ascites, instillation of methotrexate into the peritoneal cavity may slow the rate of reaccumulation of ascitic fluid

614
In the investigation of pancreatic disease
A radiological evidence of ileus in the duodenum and jejunum is a recognised feature of acute pancreatitis
B fibreoptic duodenoscopy with endoscopic retrograde cholangio-pancreatography (ERCP) is of value
C intravenous cholangiography may be of value in the diagnosis of carcinoma of the head of the pancreas
D microscopy of the stools is of more help in adults than in children
E the glucose tolerance test is typically normal in carcinoma of the pancreas

615
The following statements regarding the pancreas are correct:
A Pancreatic endocrine tissue accounts for about 10 per cent of the mass of the organ
B In about 10 per cent of individuals the main outflow of pancreatic juice enters the duodenum by a separate orifice from the common bile duct
C Pancreatic juice is hypertonic with respect to plasma
D Digestion may be impaired if the bicarbonate content of the pancreatic juice is reduced
E Maximal flow of pancreatic juice occurs one hour after a meal

616
Acute pancreatitis
A is commoner in women than in men
B is due in the majority of cases to impaction of a gall stone at the sphincter of Oddi
C arises from autodigestion of the pancreatic blood vessels and parenchyma by pancreatic enzymes
D is a recognised complication of alcoholic excess
E may complicate hypothermia

617
Recognised features of acute pancreatitis include
A an onset within 12–14 hours following the consumption of a large meal
B radiation of pain to either shoulder
C profound shock without pain
D jaundice
E severe persistent diarrhoea

618
The following statements regarding acute pancreatitis are correct:
A Rigidity and guarding of the abdominal muscles is a characteristic early feature
B The condition may simulate acute cholecystitis
C The serum amylase activity is characteristically normal within the first 12 hours following the onset of the disease
D A persistently raised serum amylase activity suggests the formation of a pseudocyst
E Hypercalcaemia occurs within a week of the onset

619
In the treatment of acute pancreatitis
A early laparotomy is mandatory
B antibiotics are contra-indicated
C morphine is likely to cause spasm of the sphincter of Oddi
D corticosteroids have no specific role
E aprotinin may be of benefit

620
Chronic pancreatitis
A may follow obstruction of a main pancreatic duct
B is a recognised complication of chronic duodenal ulcer
C when associated with haemochromatosis is characterised by intralobular fibrosis
D when due to ampullary papilloma is associated with early atrophy of the islet tissue
E is characteristically associated with a persistently elevated serum amylase activity

621
Recognised features of chronic pancreatitis include
A relief of pain by lying supine
B exacerbation of symptoms on the day after an occasion of alcoholic excess
C a reduction in salt content of the sweat
D an increase in pancreatic secretory volume
E pancreatic calcification on a plain film of the abdomen

622
In the treatment of chronic pancreatitis
A the associated diabetes mellitus will respond in most cases to treatment with an oral hypoglycaemic agent
B the presence of pancreatic cysts is a contra-indication to surgery
C a high fat diet should be recommended
D surgery should be advised if the patient is unable to give up alcohol
E the presence of stenosis of the ampulla of Vater carries a poor prognosis

623
Cystic fibrosis of the pancreas
A is an autosomal dominant disorder
B is characterised by a generalised dysfunction of mucus secreting glands
C may be complicated by right ventricular failure
D is characteristically associated with a sweat sodium concentration exceeding 80 mmol/l
E may present in the newborn with small intestinal obstruction

624
Pancreatic pseudocysts
A characteristically develop within 10 days of the onset of acute pancreatitis
B typically occupy the lesser sac
C are smaller than intrapancreatic (retention) cysts
D are associated with leucocytosis
E can hardly ever be defined by ultrasound scanning

625
Carcinoma of the pancreas
A is characteristically a scirrhous adenocarcinoma
B involves the body of the gland in the majority of cases
C is characterised by sharp spasms of epigastric pain radiating to one or other shoulder
D may present with diabetes mellitus
E may cause painless jaundice

626
The following investigations may be of diagnostic value in patients with carcinoma of the pancreas:
A barium meal
B intravenous cholangiography
C exfoliative cytology of the duodenal aspirate
D selective arteriography
E estimation of the serum amylase activity

627
The following statements regarding the small intestinal absorption of fat are correct:
A Absorption of fat takes place predominantly in the ileum
B Pancreatic lipase hydrolyses triglycerides to monoglycerides and fatty acids
C In the absorptive cell the hydrolysis of triglycerides continues
D The upper limit of normal for faecal fat excretion in patients on a normal diet is 12 g per day
E Measurement of the absorption of thiamin can be used as an indirect assessment of fat absorption

628

The following statements are correct:

A Lactose is broken down by intestinal lactase to glucose and galactose

B The glucose tolerance test is a valuable means of assessing minor degrees of carbohydrate malabsorption

C Initial digestion of dietary protein depends on gastric pepsin and pancreatic enzymes

D In health, on a normal diet, no more than 2.5 g of nitrogen is excreted in the stools each day

E Dietary vitamin B_{12} is absorbed in the lower jejunum

629

The following statements are correct:

A In Crohn's disease reabsorption of bile acids is impaired

B Colonisation of the small bowel by bacteria is a recognised cause of deconjugation of bile acids

C Intraluminal digestion may be impaired following gastro-enterostomy

D In tropical sprue the primary cause of malabsorption is impaired transport from the mucosal cell

E In steatorrhoea due to coeliac disease, the absorption of vitamins and minerals is usually normal

630

Recognised causes of intestinal malabsorption include

A giardiasis

B abdominal lymphoma

C mucosal lipase deficiency

D Polya partial gastrectomy

E interruption of the enterohepatic circulation of bile acids

631

In a patient with intestinal malabsorption

A partial villous atrophy is pathognomonic of coeliac disease

B of mild degree, bowel function may be normal

C barium follow-through characteristically shows dilated loops of small intestine with flocculation and segmentation of the contrast medium

D due to insufficiency of bile salts, the appropriate treatment is to give bile salts orally

E oral cholestyramine can be used to correct steatorrhoea

632

In coeliac disease

A the toxic agent causing mucosal damage is a polypeptide named gliadin

B the onset is typically in the middle or late teens

C there is a predisposition to the development of lymphomas of the alimentary tract

D a gluten-free diet may correct malabsorption but does not alter the histology of the intestinal mucosa

E oral corticosteroids may be beneficial in patients who fail to respond to a gluten-free diet

633

Crohn's disease

A is confined to the ileum and colon

B has a significant familial association with ankylosing spondylitis

C most commonly occurs after the age of 50

D is associated with deficiencies in delayed hypersensitivity

E is distinguished histologically from tuberculosis by the absence of caseation

634

Characteristic pathological features of Crohn's disease include

A a 'cobble-stone' mucosal pattern

B 'skip' lesions

C inflammatory changes confined to the bowel mucosa

D mesenteric lymphadenopathy

E granulomas composed of epithelioid and giant cells

635
Recognised complications of Crohn's disease include
A erythema marginatum
B iritis
C pernicious anaemia
D hydronephrosis
E perianal abscess

636
In Crohn's disease
A diarrhoea is characteristically more severe than in ulcerative colitis
B protein-losing enteropathy is a recognised complication
C passage of frank blood in the stools indicates involvement of the terminal ileum
D acute intestinal obstruction is a common complication
E the Schilling test produces a result identical to that in pernicious anaemia

637
In the investigation of Crohn's disease
A about 75 per cent of cases will show abnormalities of the caecum in barium studies
B barium enema may show abnormalities in the colon indistinguishable from those of ulcerative colitis
C the 'string sign' seen during barium follow-through examination is pathognomonic
D culture of stools characteristically yields a growth of *Strep. faecalis*
E the diagnosis may be confirmed by histological examination of a rectal biopsy

638
In the treatment of Crohn's disease
A oral cholestyramine may reduce the diarrhoea
B an elemental (no residue) diet is of particular value in patients with external fistulae for whom surgery is planned
C corticosteroids are contra-indicated in patients with active disease
D a prolonged (4-6 week) course of ampicillin may be of some benefit
E surgical bypass yields better results than resection in patients with localised disease

639
Intestinal obstruction
A is described as 'mechanical' when strangulation has occurred
B of the mechanical type may be complicated by paralytic obstruction
C can be caused by impaction of faeces in the rectum in an aged or bedridden patient
D of the paralytic type is a feature of shock
E is unlikely to be due to a hernia in an elderly patient

640
In patients with intestinal obstruction
A dehydration may occur in the absence of vomiting and diarrhoea
B renal failure is a recognised complication in the elderly
C paralytic ileus is characterised by loud borborygmi
D involving the lower small bowel vomiting may be absent
E the rectum is usually empty and collapsed

641
Peritonitis
A may result from chemical irritation
B complicating appendicitis is characteristically caused by intestinal anaerobic organisms
C now carries a very low mortality
D when due to tuberculosis is characteristically a blood-borne infection arising from a primary lung lesion
E causes abdominal rigidity which increases as paralytic ileus develops

642
The following statements are correct:
A Pelvic abscess typically presents with urinary retention
B Constipation is a characteristic early feature of pelvic abscess
C Subphrenic abscess may be associated with X-ray changes in the lung above
D Oedema over the lower ribs posteriorly is a recognised feature of subphrenic abscess
E Subphrenic abscesses are best treated conservatively

643
Acute appendicitis
A characteristically commences with pain in the right iliac fossa
B is usually associated with severe and persistent vomiting
C can be distinguished from right sided pyelonephritis by the absence of urinary symptoms
D may present with diarrhoea
E is typically associated with obstruction to the lumen of the appendix

644
The following statements are correct:
A Mild appendicitis is best treated conservatively
B Acute appendicitis is characteristically associated with rigors
C In childhood, non-specific mesenteric lymphadenitis is a recognised sequel of acute appendicitis
D Chronic appendicitis is a frequent cause of recurrent abdominal pain in young adults
E Immediate surgery is essential if there is a clearly defined appendix mass

645
The following statements regarding the aetiology of ulcerative colitis are correct:
A An abnormal immune response to faecal bacteria has been suggested
B A specific allergy to milk protein is a proven factor
C Affected patients possess a specific personality structure
D There is a significant familial association with Crohn's disease
E Secondary alactasia may cause exacerbation of the diarrhoea

646
In ulcerative colitis
A the rectum is always involved
B the inflammatory changes in the bowel are typically patchy
C pseudo-polyposis occurs as a sequel to mucosal sloughing
D the inflammatory changes characteristically extend through all layers of the bowel
E deep clefts or fissures open on to the mucosal surface

647
Recognised complications of ulcerative colitis include
A an increased incidence of carcinoma of the colon
B pyoderma gangrenosum
C arthropathy
D cholangitis
E erythema nodosum

648
In the primary management of ulcerative colitis
A administration of broad spectrum antibiotics is recommended in all patients
B a high residue diet supplemented by bran should be advised
C correction of hypokalaemia is essential
D the mouth should be inspected regularly for evidence of thrush
E the administration of codeine phosphate may precipitate an attack of toxic dilatation

649
In the treatment of ulcerative colitis
A local steroids should not be administered for longer than two weeks
B azathioprine is the drug of first choice in milder cases
C oral corticosteroids are more effective than long-acting corticotrophin injections in the treatment of a relapse
D sulphasalazine is of benefit in the prevention of relapse
E with toxic dilatation, emergency total proctocolectomy is the treatment of choice

650
Ulcerative colitis
A occurs at all ages
B has an immediate death rate of at least 40 per cent when it presents in an acute fulminating form
C is more commonly complicated by perianal fistulae than is Crohn's disease
D is much more often associated with aphthous stomatitis than is Crohn's disease
E in contrast to Crohn's disease, is not complicated by stricture formation in the chronic form

651
The following factors predispose to the development of colonic diverticula:
A a low residue diet
B congenital deficiencies in the muscular coat of the bowel
C an increased intracolonic pressure
D acquired megacolon
E spasm at the pelvirectal junction

652
Colonic diverticula
A occur most commonly in the pelvic colon
B have a well-defined muscle coat
C complicated by repeated bouts of inflammation lead to progressive dilatation of the bowel lumen
D are a recognised precursor of colonic carcinoma
E are best diagnosed by sigmoidoscopy

653
The following statements regarding carcinoma of the large intestine are correct:
A Early obstruction is characteristic of tumours of the left colon
B Only a minority of rectal tumours can be felt on digital examination
C Caecal lesions are in most cases adequately visualised during barium enema examination
D Endoscopy should be performed in all cases
E After resection, recurrence may be detected by the measurement of carcino-embryonic antigen levels

654
Carcinoma of the large intestine
A occurs in the U.K. less commonly than carcinoma of the stomach
B has a recognised association with multiple polyposis of the colon
C affects the ascending more commonly than the descending colon
D is multiple in about 2 per cent of cases
E appears in a barium enema as a filling defect or as a stricture

655
Hirschsprung's disease
A is due to congenital absence of the myenteric nerve plexus
B affects girls more commonly than boys
C characteristically presents first between the ages of 3 and 5
D is characterised by a loaded rectum on digital examination
E cannot be treated surgically

656
The following statements regarding polyps of the large intestine are correct:
A Those larger than 1 cm in diameter are probably malignant
B Multiple polyposis is transmitted as an autosomal recessive trait
C In multiple polyposis colectomy should not be advised unless at least one of the polyps has shown malignant change
D They are a recognised cause of intussusception
E Benign polyps occur less commonly than myomas of the large bowel

657
The small intestine is characteristically involved in
A cholera
B bacillary dysentery
C strongyloidiasis
D ancylostomiasis
E amoebic dysentery

658
Specific antimicrobial therapy is routinely indicated in
A 'travellers' diarrhoea'
B Esch. coli gastroenteritis
C bacillary dysentery due to Shigella sonnei
D giardiasis
E mild salmonella food poisoning

659
The following statements regarding vascular disorders of the alimentary tract are correct:
A Occlusion of the superior mesenteric artery is characterised by sudden severe abdominal pain, vomiting and watery diarrhoea
B Occlusion of the inferior mesenteric artery may simulate diverticular disease
C Malabsorption is a recognised complication of chronic ischaemia of the bowel
D An underlying cause can be found in the great majority of patients over the age of 50 suffering from ischaemic colitis
E Chronic ischaemia of the bowel may lead to stricture formation

660
Characteristic features of the irritable bowel syndrome include
A an obsession with bowel function
B an empty rectum on digital examination
C the passage of hard stools accompanied by mucus
D morning vomiting
E nocturnal diarrhoea

CHAPTER NINE

661
In the normal liver
A the portal tracts are separated from the liver lobule by the space of Disse
B the sinusoids convey blood from the hepatic vein to the portal vein
C total liver blood flow is approximately 500 ml per minute
D the hepatic artery arises directly from the aorta
E bile canaliculi form networks between the hepatocytes

662
On examination of the liver
A the normal upper border follows the line of the right seventh rib
B the normal lower margin crosses the epigastrium midway between the xiphisternum and the umbilicus
C percussion is of value in revealing a small liver
D an arterial bruit may be heard in acute alcoholic hepatitis
E the venous hum audible between the xiphisternum and the umbilicus is characteristic of a hepatoma

663
The following statements about protein metabolism are correct:
A The components of the complement system are synthesised in the liver
B Alpha-fetoprotein is normally only made by the liver prior to and shortly after birth
C Alpha$_1$-antitrypsin is synthesised exclusively in the lungs
D The electrophoretic pattern of normal plasma is largely determined by liver function
E Urea synthesis occurring as a result of aminoacid deamination takes place solely in the liver

664
In the metabolism of lipids
A newly synthesised lipid molecules are combined with specific apoproteins to form lipoproteins in the liver
B lipoprotein lipase facilitates the uptake of dietary triglyceride by the liver
C triglycerides synthesised in the liver are transported by low density lipoproteins (ß)
D the serum lipid concentration falls in biliary obstruction
E the liver is the main site of cholesterol synthesis

665
Bilirubin
A is derived exclusively from haemoglobin breakdown
B in the unconjugated form is carried in plasma bound to a ß-globulin
C is conjugated in the microsomes of the hepatocytes
D in its water soluble form is re-absorbed in small quantities in the small intestine
E is normally excreted mainly in the form of stercobilinogen and stercobilin

666
The following statements are correct:
A In the gut the majority of bile acids are reabsorbed in the terminal ileum
B Deoxycholic acid is formed from chenodeoxycholic acid in the colon
C The majority of secondary bile acids are excreted in the faeces
D The maintenance of the micellar state depends principally on the cholesterol content of the micelles
E Excess of bile acids in the colon is a recognised cause of diarrhoea

667
Conjugated bilirubin
A is not detectable in the urine of normal persons
B is excreted in the urine in parallel with urobilinogen in viral hepatitis
C is present in normal serum in higher concentration than unconjugated bilirubin
D is present in excess in the serum in haemolytic anaemia
E is excreted by active transport into the bile

668
Serum transferase activity
A is a measure of the integrity of the liver cells
B is not increased in obstructive jaundice
C does not increase in viral hepatitis until jaundice is evident
D changes in chronic liver disease are of prognostic value
E characteristically shows an increase of at least tenfold in acute alcoholic hepatitis

669
In tests of liver function using serum
A alanine aminotransferase is a more specific indicator of hepatocellular damage than aspartate amino-transferase
B elevation of the alkaline phosphatase activity during normal pregnancy indicates hepatic cholestasis
C gamma-glutamyl transpeptidase activity is typically reduced in acute alcoholic hepatitis
D the albumin concentration falls early in acute viral hepatitis
E the hyperglobulinaemia of cirrhosis reflects liver cell damage

670
In the investigation of liver disease
A a rise of the serum IgA concentration is characteristic of primary biliary cirrhosis
B the finding of monoclonal gammopathy is of serious prognostic significance in portal cirrhosis
C changes in prothrombin time occur rapidly after liver cell damage
D progressive increase in prothrombin time during the course of acute hepatitis indicates a worsening prognosis
E bromsulphthalein excretion remains a valid test of liver function in the presence of jaundice

671
The hepatitis B surface antigen (HBsAg)
A can be detected in the blood during the prodromal phase of acute type B hepatitis
B persists in the blood of approximately 25 per cent of patients following an episode of acute type B hepatitis
C is a recognised finding in the blood of some patients with hepatoma
D is found in the blood of apparently healthy individuals more commonly in Europe and North America than in the tropics
E is attached to a virus which causes chronic hepatitis

672
In the investigation of suspected liver disease
A the diagnosis of malignancy is more often missed by percutaneous needle biopsy than is chronic persistent hepatitis
B the anterior surface is not normally visible during peritoneoscopy
C ultrasound scanning will not differentiate between a solid and a cystic intrahepatic mass
D a normal radioisotope scan reliably excludes liver disease
E a protein content in excess of 30g/l in ascitic fluid is usual in hepatic vein thrombosis

673
Haemolytic jaundice in the adult
A becomes clinically evident when the serum bilirubin concentration exceeds 50 μmol/l (3mg/100ml)
B is typically associated with a serum bilirubin between 85 and 170 μmol/l (5–10mg/100ml)
C is associated with the passage of urine which darkens on standing
D is, in most patients, associated with splenomegaly
E is characterised by passage of pale stools

674
The following statements are correct:
A In hepatocellular jaundice the blood concentrations of both unconjugated and conjugated bilirubin increase
B Alcohol is a recognised cause of jaundice due to widespread small duct obstruction
C Rigors occurring in association with obstructive jaundice are characteristic of hepatic metastases
D Long-standing obstructive jaundice may be complicated by bone pain
E A palpable gallbladder in the presence of obstructive jaundice suggests impaction of a gallstone in the common bile duct

675
Characteristic features of Gilbert's syndrome include
A inheritance as sex-linked recessive trait
B unconjugated hyperbilirubinaemia
C elevation of serum transferase activity
D reduced serum haptoglobin concentration
E diminution of jaundice after oral administration of phenobarbitone

676
The following agents are recognised causes of acute parenchymal liver disease:
A Epstein-Barr virus
B *Coxiella burneti*
C chlorpromazine
D methyldopa
E *Toxoplasma gondii*

677
Cholestatic jaundice is a recognised unwanted effect of therapy with
A rifampicin
B salicylates
C oestrogen-containing oral contraceptives
D C-17 alkyl substituted testosterones
E phenobarbitone

678
The histological changes of viral hepatitis include
A sparing of the centrilobular areas
B infiltration of lobules with polymorphonuclear leucocytes
C fatty degeneration
D eosinophilic (Councilman) bodies
E collapse of the reticulin framework

679
The following statements concerning type A hepatitis are correct:
A The virus causing the disease can be isolated by culture of faeces
B A carrier state for type A hepatitis has not yet been identified
C Outbreaks have been traced to ingestion of contaminated shellfish
D A polymorphonuclear leucocytosis in the prodromal phase is characteristic
E the appearance of cholestasis in a liver biopsy carries a bad prognosis

680
The following statements are correct:
A The post-hepatitis syndrome is due to persisting viraemia with focal hepatic necrosis
B Pancytopenia may occur some months after recovery from acute type A hepatitis
C Patients travelling to endemic hepatitis A areas may be fully protected by a vaccine
D Those who have been in contact with a patient suffering from type A hepatitis may be protected by injection of gamma globulin
E In young adults, acute type A hepatitis carries a mortality of less than 1 per cent

681
Type B hepatitis virus
A can be transmitted to guinea pigs
B may be transmitted by intravenous infusion of human albumin
C causes a more severe illness than Type A virus
D should be suspected as the causative agent if arthritis complicates an episode of acute hepatitis
E infection may be prevented by injection of standard gamma globulin

682
Characteristic features of fulminant hepatic failure include
A hepatic encephalopathy
B massive hepatomegaly
C rapidly progressive jaundice
D foetor hepaticus
E splenomegaly

683
In patients with fulminant hepatic failure
A the serum transferase activity rises throughout the illness
B only a minority of those who survive regain normal hepatic function
C renal failure is a recognised complication
D hypoglycaemia is a typical feature
E leucopenia is characteristic

684
In a jaundiced patient the following features would suggest large duct biliary obstruction rather than acute viral hepatitis:
A marked pruritus
B a serum alkaline phosphatase activity of 150 u/l (30 KA units/100ml)
C leucocytosis
D a palpable gall bladder
E tenderness in the right hypochondrium

685
In the management of a patient with acute parenchymal liver disease
A complete bed rest until jaundice has disappeared is mandatory
B a high calorie diet is desirable
C protein intake should be restricted
D corticosteroids should be avoided
E alcohol may be taken once the appetite returns

686
The management of a patient with fulminant hepatic failure should include
A a protein free diet
B sedation with barbiturates if the patient is restless
C oral lactulose
D serial blood glucose estimations
E correction of potassium deficiency

687
Hepatic cirrhosis
A is cryptogenic in 30 per cent of cases
B is less likely to occur in association
   with a regular daily intake of alcohol
   than with episodic drinking
C may follow severe type B hepatitis
   within a few months of the acute
   illness
D is a recognised complication of
   methyldopa therapy
E is a recognised complication of
   kwashiorkor

688
**Characteristic histological features of
chronic aggressive hepatitis include**
A sparing of the portal tracts
B distortion of the lobular architecture
C a mononuclear cell infiltrate affecting
   predominantly the centrilobular region
D 'piecemeal' necrosis
E diffuse fatty change throughout the
   liver

689
Active chronic hepatitis
A affects predominantly males over the
   age of 30
B in the female is characteristically
   associated with menorrhagia
C has an acute onset in about a quarter
   of the cases
D is characteristically associated with
   spider telangiectasia
E should not be diagnosed in the absence
   of jaundice

690
**Recognised associations of active
chronic hepatitis include**
A Sjögren's syndrome
B migrating polyarthritis
C Hashimoto's thyroiditis
D Coombs'-positive haemolytic anaemia
E lymphadenopathy

691
In patients with active chronic hepatitis
A the clinical course is marked by
   exacerbations and remissions
B clinical deterioration is likely to be
   more rapid when the HBs antigen is
   present in the blood
C a confident diagnosis can be made by
   liver biopsy within two months of the
   onset
D circulating smooth muscle antibodies
   can be detected in the majority of
   patients
E corticosteroids offer no therapeutic
   benefit

692
**Recognised features of hepatic cirrhosis
in the adult include**
A increasing hepatomegaly as the disease
   progresses
B parotid gland enlargement
C gaseous abdominal distension
D macrocytosis
E massive splenomegaly

693
In patients with hepatic cirrhosis
A the presence of oesophago-gastric
   varices establishes a diagnosis of portal
   hypertension
B increasing jaundice implies progressing
   liver failure
C a reduced glomerular filtration rate
   contributes to the development of
   ascites
D a reduced peripheral blood flow is
   characteristic
E central cyanosis is a recognised feature

694
In hepatic cirrhosis
A unilateral gynaecomastia is a
   recognised feature
B libido is reduced in the male but
   increased in the female
C hyperpigmentation is due to iron
   deposition in the skin
D there is a statistically highly significant
   association with Dupuytren's
   contracture
E there is a low grade pyrexia, in the
   absence of infection, in about a third of
   patients

695

Hepatic encephalopathy may be precipitated in a cirrhotic patient by
A a surgical operation
B oral neomycin
C hypokalaemia
D constipation
E the administration of barbiturates

696

In the investigation of a patient with hepatic cirrhosis
A excessive urobilinogenuria is a recognised feature
B the serum transferase activity is characteristically increased at least ten-fold
C serial estimation of the serum alkaline phosphatase activity is of prognostic value
D the bromsulphthalein test should be interpreted with caution in the presence of hypoalbuminaemia
E HBs antigenaemia is a recognised finding

697

Primary biliary cirrhosis
A is associated with pruritus only when jaundice is clinically evident
B is characterised by recurrent rigors
C may be complicated by bone pain in the later stages
D is associated with xanthomatous deposits in the majority of patients
E is typically associated with a positive antimitochondrial antibody test

698

In the management of patients with hepatic cirrhosis
A successful treatment of ascites improves the prognosis
B vitamin supplements should be prescribed routinely
C in the absence of cholestasis dietary fat need not be restricted
D frusemide is the drug of first choice in the treatment of ascites
E gynaecomastia may occur as a complication of therapy

699

In the management of bleeding from oesophageal varices in a patient with cirrhosis
A intravenous vasopressin may promote haemostasis by reducing portal venous pressure
B endoscopy is contra-indicated
C the Minnesota tube allows secretions to be aspirated from the upper oesophagus
D an emergency portal-systemic shunt operation is the treatment of choice if bleeding continues
E oesophageal transection may be the only effective way to stop bleeding

700

Contraindications to a portal-systemic shunt operation include
A a serum albumin concentration below 35 g/l
B ascites
C a serum bilirubin concentration of 70µmol/l (4mg/100ml)
D age over 70 years
E splenomegaly

701

In patients with chronic cholestasis
A pruritus may be relieved by administration of cholestyramine
B administration of norethandrolone for pruritus is likely to increase jaundice
C osteomalacia is a recognised complication
D due to primary biliary cirrhosis, corticosteroids are beneficial
E continuous oral antibiotic therapy is indicated if cholangitis is present

702

In hepatolenticular degeneration (Wilson's disease)
A cirrhosis may occur in the absence of any neurological abnormality
B Kayser-Fleischer rings do not occur unless abnormal neurological signs are present
C the onset may mimic that of viral hepatitis
D fulminant hepatic failure is a recognised complication
E jaundice is occasionally haemolytic in origin

703
Recognised causes of portal hypertension include
A primary biliary cirrhosis
B hepatic venous outflow obstruction (Budd-Chiari syndrome)
C splenic vein thrombosis
D schistosomiasis
E exposure to vinyl chloride

704
Hepatic venous outflow obstruction (Budd-Chiari syndrome)
A may complicate polycythaemia rubra vera
B may be treated successfully by anticoagulants
C results in centrilobular congestion
D typically has an insidious onset
E causes ascites

705
The following statements are correct:
A Polycystic disease of the liver is associated with polycystic renal disease in 90 per cent of cases
B Congenital hepatic fibrosis is a recognised cause of portal hypertension in childhood
C Cerebral arterial aneurysms are a recognised association of polycystic liver disease
D Porphyria cutanea tarda is a recognised complication of hepatoma
E Splenomegaly is present in most patients with secondary carcinoma of the liver

706
Primary hepatocellular carcinoma
A occurs more commonly in females than in males
B may be due to the ingestion of aflatoxin-contaminated food in tropical countries
C may be associated with an audible bruit over the liver
D can be confidently diagnosed if alpha-fetoprotein is present in the blood
E may be complicated by polycythaemia

707
Regarding the gall bladder and bile ducts
A the common bile duct is formed from the junction of the right and left hepatic ducts
B the lumen of the common bile duct is widest distally
C the common bile and pancreatic ducts enter the duodenal lumen separately in the majority of individuals
D the intraluminal pressure in the common bile duct is probably maintained principally by the choledochal sphincter (sphincter of Oddi)
E the gall bladder is innervated principally by sympathetic nerves

708
The following statements are correct:
A Cholecystokinin causes contraction of the choledochal sphincter
B Regular peristalsis occurs in the common bile duct
C Morphine causes relaxation of the choledochal sphincter
D Acetylcholine causes contraction of the gall bladder
E There is normally no reflux of bile into the pancreatic duct

709
Regarding the radiology of the gall bladder
A at least 50 per cent of all stones are radio-opaque
B gas in the biliary tree is a sign of a fistulous communication with the intestine
C the normal gall bladder can be seen to contract in response to a fatty meal during oral cholecystography
D failure of visualisation of the gall bladder during oral cholecystography may be due to pyloric stenosis
E percutaneous transhepatic cholangiography is contra-indicated in a deeply jaundiced patient

710
Gallstones
A occur more frequently in the Bantu population than in white South Africans
B contain cholesterol in over 75 per cent of cases
C are prone to occur when cholesterol is precipitated from bile by an excess of bile acids
D are a recognised unwanted effect of the long term use of oestrogen containing oral contraceptives
E are more likely to occur in the presence of infection of the gall bladder than when this is absent

711
The following statements are correct:
A Acute cholecystitis does not occur in the absence of gallstones
B Acute cholecystitis typically follows obstruction of the gall bladder neck or the cystic duct
C Culture of gall bladder contents 72 hours after the onset of symptoms of cholecystitis is usually sterile
D If a patient with acute cholecystitis is given morphine for the relief of pain, it is advisable to give atropine simultaneously
E In the treatment of gallstones, chenodeoxycholic acid is more effective in dissolving radiopaque than radiolucent stones

712
Acute cholecystitis
A has decreased in incidence in patients under the age of 40 in the last 20 years
B is commonly accompanied by leucopenia
C may be associated with a rise in the serum amylase activity
D may mimic retro-caecal appendicitis
E is best treated by emergency cholecystectomy

713
Recognised complications of gallstone disease include
A acute pancreatitis
B intestinal obstruction
C ascending cholangitis
D xanthomatous deposits in the skin
E carcinoma of the gallbladder

714
The following statements are correct:
A Cholesterolosis of the gallbladder leads to failure of concentration of the radio-opaque medium during oral cholecystography
B Adenomyomatosis of the gall bladder produces a filling defect in the gall bladder during oral cholecystography
C 'Biliary dyskinesia' is best treated by choledochoduodenostomy
D Secondary biliary cirrhosis is a recognised complication of sclerosing cholangitis
E Choledochal cysts rarely present clinically over the age of 30

715
Carcinoma of the gall bladder
A shows a peak incidence in men between the ages of 40 and 50
B is typically anaplastic in type
C is associated with jaundice in less than 10 per cent of patients
D is associated with calcification of the organ on abdominal X-ray
E is usually inoperable

716
Cholangiocarcinoma is
A associated with hepatic cirrhosis
B an adenocarcinoma
C associated with obstructive jaundice
D slow growing
E typically associated with the presence of alpha-fetoprotein in the blood

CHAPTER TEN

717
Regarding the normal kidney
A each is composed of approximately 100 000 nephrons
B afferent arterioles arising from the renal artery give rise to the glomerular capillaries
C the afferent arterioles supply blood directly to the proximal and distal convoluted tubules
D the medulla is supplied by efferent arterioles which arise from glomeruli in the deeper regions of the cortex
E the hydrostatic pressure within the glomerular capillaries is approximately 80 mm Hg

718
The following statements regarding the normal kidney are correct:
A The juxtaglomerular apparatus is composed of specialised cells in the walls of the proximal convoluted tubule and the efferent arteriole
B About one-third of the water filtered by the glomerulus is re-absorbed by the proximal tubule
C Absorption of water from the distal tubules is influenced chiefly by vasopressin
D The glomerular filtrate contains approximately 0.2 g protein/l
E The kidney is the main source of erythropoietin

719

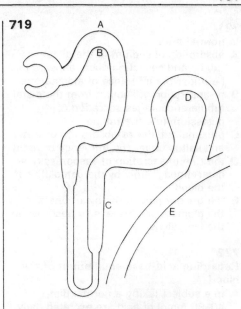

The diagram is of a single nephron. At the sites identified the following functions take place:
A active potassium secretion
B active sodium re-absorption
C passive chloride re-absorption
D potassium re-absorption
E ammonia secretion

720
The following functional exchanges take place in the collecting duct of the nephron:
A active secretion of potassium
B secretion of hydrogen ion
C bicarbonate secretion
D passive re-absorption of water
E passive re-absorption of sodium

721
In normal man
A absorption of sodium in the distal tubule and collecting ducts appears to be under the influence of aldosterone
B re-absorption of sodium from the distal tubule encourages secretion of potassium into the tubule
C proximal tubular re-absorption of water and salt is under the influence of renin
D the rate of secretion of vasopressin is determined mainly by the osmolality of the blood
E the greater part of the bicarbonate in the glomerular filtrate is re-absorbed in the loop of Henle

722
Regarding acid-base equilibrium of the blood
A in a subject taking a normal diet, 40–80 mmol of acid are excreted daily into the urine
B on a vegetarian diet, tubular secretion of ammonium ions is increased
C. carbonic anhydrase within the renal tubular cell plays a fundamental role in maintaining homeostasis
D anions of inorganic and organic acids are excreted in the urine largely as ammonium salts
E hydrogen ions in the urine are buffered both by disodium hydrogen phosphate and ammonia

723
Congenital or acquired abnormalities of renal tubular transport may result in
A increased retention of phosphate
B glycosuria
C increased retention of water
D abnormal urinary loss of amino-acids
E abnormal urinary loss of potassium

724
Renal tubular acidosis
A results in a defect in the power to acidify the urine
B is a recognised complication of chronic pyelonephritis
C is a recognised feature of Wilson's disease
D is apt to lead to hyperkalaemia
E may result from the administration of degraded tetracycline

725
The following statements concerning the kidney are correct:
A The juxtaglomerular apparatus secretes angiotensin I
B The normal 24 h urinary excretion of protein is approximately 50 mg
C The organ is responsible for the formation of 1,25 dihydroxycholecalciferol
D A normal individual must excrete approximately 1500 ml urine daily to maintain the *milieu intérieur* of the body if the diet is normal
E A low protein and salt diet leads to an increased urinary output

726
Oliguria is
A defined as a daily urinary output of less than one litre
B a recognised feature of untreated cardiac failure
C a characteristic feature of potassium depletion
D a recognised consequence of hypotension
E a constant feature of chronic renal disease with uraemia

727
Urinary specific gravity
A is a measure of the quantity of solids in solution
B is increased approximately three times as much by urea as by a similar quantity of protein
C is independent of the nature and quantity of food eaten
D after deprivation of fluid in normal individuals for 20 hours in temperate climates does not exceed 1.025
E in health is influenced mainly by the urinary excretion of ammonium salts

728
The following statements concerning renal function are correct:
A In health, no free hydrogen ion is excreted in the urine
B Infections of the urinary tract with *Esch. Coli* cause the urine to become alkaline
C The concept of renal clearance is expressed by the equation $C = \dfrac{P}{UV}$
D Measurement of the renal clearance of endogenous urea in the normal individual gives a reliable estimate of glomerular filtration rate
E The blood urea concentration does not rise above the accepted normal maximum until renal function is reduced by at least 50 per cent

729
Proteinuria in excess of 3 g/day is a recognised feature of
A minimal lesion glomerulonephritis
B heart failure
C renal vein thrombosis
D polycystic renal disease
E chronic pyelonephritis

730
Haematuria, macroscopic or microscopic, is an expected finding in
A membranous glomerulonephritis
B renal amyloidosis
C malignant hypertension
D renal infarction
E infective endocarditis

731
Red or pink colouration of the urine, in the absence of red cells visible microscopically, is a recognised feature of
A haemoglobinuria
B the presence of phenolphthalein in an acid urine
C ingestion of beetroot
D urine passed some hours previously by a patient with acute intermittent porphyria
E benign prostatic hypertrophy

732
Proliferative glomerulonephritis
A is due to the deposition of antigen—antibody complexes on the endothelial side of the glomerular basement membrane
B follows infection with haemolytic streptococci more often than with other organisms
C may be associated with haemoptysis
D carries a poorer prognosis in children than in adults
E does not follow viral infections

733
Pathological renal changes in proliferative glomerulonephritis include
A accumulation of eosinophils in the glomerular tuft
B epithelial crescent formation
C proliferation of mesangial cells
D progressive glomerular fibrosis
E intravascular glomerular thrombosis

734
The following statements regarding proliferative glomerulonephritis are correct:
A A rise in serum complement (C3) occurs in poststreptococcal glomerulonephritis
B Only a minority of patients show a rise in diastolic blood pressure during the acute phase
C Impairment of the concentrating power of the urine is a characteristic early finding
D Despite an apparent return to normal health after the acute episode, renal failure may develop many years later
E In the acute phase, death from acute cardiac failure may occur within a few days of the onset

735
In the treatment of acute proliferative glomerulonephritis
A dietary protein restriction accelerates the healing process
B fluid intake should be restricted while oedema is present
C salt restriction is seldom necessary
D corticosteroids are of proven benefit
E no therapy is required for hypertension in the majority of patients

736
Membranous glomerulonephritis
A is characterised by diffuse hyaline thickening of the glomerular capillary walls
B shows similar mesangial cell proliferation to that seen in proliferative glomerulonephritis
C leads to a reduction in the permeability of the glomerular basement membrane
D is not preceded by any recognisable infection
E is commonly associated with a raised plasma cholesterol concentration

737
Glomerular disease caused by immune complexes is a recognised complication of
A systemic lupus erythematosus
B polyarteritis nodosa
C lymphoma
D acute pyelonephritis
E staphylococcal infection

738
Features of minimal lesion glomerulonephritis include
A early impairment of glomerular filtration rate
B impaired ability to concentrate the urine
C spontaneous recovery within a few weeks in the majority of cases
D a favourable response to corticosteroids
E loss of up to 3 g of protein in the urine daily

739
The following statements regarding glomerulonephritis are correct:
A In minimal lesion glomerulonephritis, abnormalities of glomerular structure are revealed only by the electron microscope
B IgE is implicated in the pathogenesis of minimal lesion glomerulonephritis
C There is a recognised association between antibodies to type B hepatitis virus and glomerulonephritis
D Membranous glomerulonephritis affects predominantly children and adults under the age of 30
E A relative increase of serum $\alpha_2$globulin occurs in both minimal lesion and membranous glomerulonephritis

740
In the treatment of the nephrotic syndrome
A frusemide is contra-indicated
B spironolactone may be of value if hypokalaemia is present
C a high protein diet should be given if the blood urea concentration is not elevated
D cyclophosphamide is the treatment of choice for membranous glomerulonephritis
E drastic salt restriction may produce dramatic results

741
Chronic glomerulonephritis
A is associated with a reduction in peripelvic fat
B more commonly follows membranous than minimal lesion glomerulonephritis
C frequently presents with no previous history of renal disease
D typically shows a reduction in renal cortical tissue on histological examination
E is associated with large, pale kidneys

742
Recognised clinical features of chronic glomerulonephritis include
A macrocytic anaemia
B bone pain
C Kussmaul's respiration
D polyuria
E peripheral neuropathy

743
Characteristic biochemical features of chronic glomerulonephritis include
A alkalosis
B hypercalcaemia
C impaired ability of the kidneys to concentrate or dilute urine
D phosphate retention
E heavy proteinuria (more than 4 g/24 h)

744
In the treatment of chronic glomerulonephritis
A fluid restriction should be rigidly enforced
B the carbohydrate content of the diet should be restricted
C in the absence of cardiac failure, oedema or hypertension, salt restriction is contra-indicated
D intercurrent infection should not be treated with tetracycline
E parenteral iron is the treatment of choice for the associated anaemia

745
Features of chronic glomerulonephritis that point to a bad prognosis include
A granular casts in the urinary deposit
B papilloedema
C spontaneous haemorrhage
D enterocolitis
E dehydration

746
In renal transplantation for chronic renal failure
A there is an overall survival rate of 50 per cent after ten years
B HLA compatibility is only important in the case of cadaver transplants
C a kidney from a healthy twin offers the best prospects
D immunosuppressive drugs are not free of complications
E the need is increasing in view of the poor results of intermittent dialysis

747
Regarding urinary infection
A the great majority of patients with recurrent lower urinary tract infection subsequently develop deterioration of renal function
B acute pyelonephritis is characterised by inflammation of the parenchyma and the pelvis of the kidney
C acute pyelonephritis is invariably bilateral
D rigors are a feature of acute pyelonephritis
E in infants, acute pyelonephritis may present with febrile convulsions

748
The following lesions are recognised as predisposing to acute pyelonephritis:
A prostatic enlargement
B cervical prolapse
C ureterovesical reflux
D renal calculi
E infective endocarditis

749
During pregnancy
A atonia of the ureters predisposes to acute pyelonephritis
B asymptomatic bacteriuria is present in approximately 20 per cent of all patients during the early months
C suppressive chemotherapy in patients with asymptomatic bacteriuria seldom prevents the development of acute symptoms
D co-trimoxazole is the drug of choice for the treatment of acute urinary infections
E motile gram-negative bacilli found on microscopy of a midstream urine sample of acid pH may be assumed to be *Esch. coli*

750
Recognised features of acute pyelonephritis with cystitis include
A leucopenia
B strangury
C necrosis of the papillae (acute necrotising papillitis)
D oedema which obliterates the normal hollow in the loin
E septicaemia

751
Chronic pyelonephritis
A is more commonly the result of proteus infection than infection with *Esch. coli*
B is a recognised complication of multiple sclerosis
C shows sparing of the renal cortex when the kidney is examined microscopically
D may present with the chance finding of hypertension
E may be complicated by pyonephrosis

752
The following statements regarding chronic pyelonephritis are correct:
A There is a recognised association between this condition and nephrocalcinosis
B The infecting organism is more easily eradicated than in acute pyelonephritis
C The prognosis is poor in paraplegic patients
D The condition is a recognised cause of excessive salt loss
E Underlying analgesic nephropathy should be excluded

753
The following statements are correct:
A In acute cystitis there is typically considerable systemic disturbance
B The 'urethral syndrome' occurs predominantly in males
C Conjunctivitis is a recognised association of urethritis
D A predisposing cause for recurrent lower urinary tract infections is found in the majority of female patients
E The passage of grossly blood-stained urine is a recognised feature of acute cystitis

754
In renal tuberculosis
A pain in the loin is the most common presenting feature
B the renal pelvis is typically affected before the cortex
C sterile pyuria is a characteristic finding
D prednisone given concurrently with chemotherapy may prevent the development of ureteric stenosis
E nephrectomy is contra-indicated

755
Recognised causes of acute renal failure include
A malignant hypertension
B systemic lupus erythematosus
C eclampsia
D disseminated intravascular coagulation
E acute circulatory failure

756
The following statements are correct:
A Prerenal uraemia due to renal ischaemia does not occur in the absence of systemic hypotension
B Incompatible blood transfusion is a recognised cause of prerenal uraemia
C Acute tubular necrosis is characterised by the passage of urine of high specific gravity
D Cephaloridine therapy may cause acute tubular necrosis
E Intraglomerular coagulation is a recognised feature of severe renal ischaemia

757
In the treatment of the oliguric phase of acute renal failure
A surgical renal decapsulation is of value
B in the absence of fever, diarrhoea or vomiting, fluid intake should be limited to 600 ml per day plus a further volume of fluid equivalent to the amount of urine passed
C dietary protein should be restricted to 40 g/day
D hyperkalaemia may be reduced by the use of an oral sodium or calcium charged resin
E a high carbohydrate intake should be encouraged

758
Haemodialysis during the oliguric phase of acute renal failure
A does not obviate the need for fluid restriction
B allows a more liberal dietary protein intake
C is preferable to peritoneal dialysis in the treatment of adults
D is of particular value when the patient has suffered massive tissue damage
E may be required daily for several weeks before renal function returns

759
During the diuretic (recovery) phase of uncomplicated acute renal failure
A the blood urea falls as soon as diuresis commences
B the daily protein intake may be increased
C salt supplements should be avoided
D oral potassium supplements may be required
E fluid restriction should be maintained

760
The following statements are correct:
A In the presence of two functioning kidneys unilateral ureteric obstruction does not cause uraemia
B Anuria is less common in postrenal uraemia than in acute tubular necrosis
C In a patient with acute renal failure, the past history of renal colic favours a diagnosis of postrenal uraemia
D In postrenal uraemia surgical treatment to relieve obstruction should be delayed until the blood urea starts to fall
E Retrograde pyelography is contra-indicated in postrenal uraemia

761
Obstruction of the urinary tract
A predisposes to stone formation
B at the lower end of the ureter causes hydronephrosis before hydro-ureter occurs
C is a recognised complication of retroperitoneal fibrosis
D when supravesical is more likely to be associated with renal colic when the obstruction is gradual in onset than when it occurs suddenly
E is seldom associated with haematuria when the obstruction is supravesical

762
Recognised factors predisposing to renal stone formation include
A urinary infection
B prolonged immobilisation
C gout
D hypoparathyroidism
E renal tubular acidosis

763
Regarding renal calculi and nephrocalcinosis
A less than 75 per cent of renal stones contain calcium
B the most common symptom of stone in the kidney is renal colic
C nephrocalcinosis characteristically causes an intermittent dull pain in the loin
D the majority of renal calculi in the United Kingdom occur in elderly women
E renal calculi may remain asymptomatic for many years

764
The pain of renal colic
A radiates from the loin in the first lumbar dermatome
B is typically associated with pallor and sweating
C is characterised by pain which comes and goes every few minutes
D when due to a ureteric calculus is associated with microscopic or macroscopic haematuria
E is best treated by regular administration of salicylates

765
In the treatment of renal calculi
A urgent surgical intervention is necessary if anuria occurs in a patient with renal colic
B the urine should be alkalinised in patients with phosphatic calculi
C cellulose phosphate taken orally may be of value in preventing recurrent stone formation in idiopathic hypercalciuria
D the use of allopurinol in the treatment of gout increases the liability to the production of urate stones
E bendrofluazide reduces urinary calcium excretion

766
The adult variety of polycystic renal disease
A is inherited as an autosomal recessive trait
B has a recognised association with cystic liver
C is characteristically unilateral
D may be found during infancy
E may cause haematuria

767
Analgesic nephropathy
A is caused only by phenacetin
B occurs more frequently in men than women
C may present with features of recurrent urinary tract infection
D may be complicated by acute papillary necrosis
E has a recognised association with transitional cell carcinoma of the renal pelvis

768
Recognised features of renal carcinoma include
A continued fever
B polycythaemia
C an avascular filling defect in the kidney on aortography
D metastasis to bone
E renal colic

769
Carcinoma of the bladder
A is typically of squamous cell type
B is a recognised sequel to chronic exposure to aniline
C typically presents with frequency and nocturia
D is unresponsive to radiotherapy
E may lead to obstructive uropathy

770
In patients with benign prostatic hypertrophy
A haematuria is a recognised presenting symptom
B the peak incidence is in the sixth decade of life
C the prostate gland may feel normal on rectal examination
D acute urinary retention may be precipitated by cardiac failure
E there is typically increased androgen secretion

771
Regarding testicular tumours
A testicular pain is a prominent feature of seminoma
B teratoma produces uniform enlargement of the testis
C gynaecomastia is a recognised complication of teratoma
D seminomas are more radiosensitive than teratomas
E the diagnosis of teratoma may be confirmed by estimating urinary or serum gonadotrophin concentrations

CHAPTER ELEVEN

772
Hypothalamic substances have been identified which
A stimulate the release of corticotrophin
B stimulate the release of thyroid stimulating hormone
C inhibit the secretion of luteinising hormone
D inhibit the secretion of growth hormone
E release the secretion of melanocyte stimulating hormones

773
Acromegaly
A affects skin as well as bone
B causes cardiac enlargement
C is a recognised cause of glycosuria
D is associated with suppression of growth hormone secretion in the course of a standard glucose tolerance test
E results from hypersecretion of basophil cells in the anterior pituitary

774
The following statements about pituitary tumours are correct:
A Chromophobe adenomas are typically associated with hypopituitarism
B Basophil tumours produce local pressure effects early
C Suprasellar calcification suggests the presence of a craniopharyngioma
D A visual field defect is a contra-indication to surgical treatment
E They may cause disturbances of sleep

775
In a case of dwarfism
A the finding of hypertension may give a clue to a possible cause
B a pituitary tumour is the most likely cause
C achondroplasia can be excluded if there is normal development of the trunk
D a prominent abdomen is a sure indication of cretinism
E the family history is particularly important

776
Hypopituitarism
A in spite of improved obstetrical care, is still most commonly due to post-partum haemorrhage
B may be caused by sarcoidosis
C usually results in loss of weight
D is more likely to cause loss of axillary and pubic hair than is anorexia nervosa
E is unlikely to cause severe electrolyte changes on account of continued function of the glomerulosa layer of the adrenal cortex

777
Diabetes insipidus
A is a recognised consequence of encephalitis
B may result in the passage of more than 20 litres of urine in 24 hours
C is easy to differentiate from hysterical polydipsia
D is best controlled by carbamazepine
E is always responsive to the administration of desmopressin

778
The thyroid gland
A is separated from the recurrent laryngeal nerves only by its fibrous sheath
B has a meagre blood supply except when thyrotoxicosis is present
C produces two bipeptides which are normally stored in the colloid vesicles
D is stimulated directly by a hypothalamic hormone without pituitary intervention
E does not produce calcitonin unless there is a medullary carcinoma of the gland

779
Thyrotoxicosis can
A occur in the absence of clinically detectable enlargement of the thyroid gland
B be excluded in a patient who is gaining weight
C cause atrial fibrillation
D cause capillary pulsation
E result in stunting of growth if it occurs before puberty

780
In the investigation of a patient with suspected thyrotoxicosis
A the effective thyroxine ratio (ETR) is unreliable if contraceptive pills are being taken
B a recent barium meal interferes with the interpretation of protein bound iodine (PBI) estimation
C the total serum thyroxine is not influenced by exogenous iodine
D the in vivo uptake of radioactive iodine by the thyroid gland is independent of the oral intake of iodine
E the TRH stimulation test is of little or no value in diagnosing T3 thyrotoxicosis

781
In the treatment of thyrotoxicosis
A potassium perchlorate is less likely than carbimazole to induce blood dyscrasia
B carbimazole blocks the organic binding of iodine to tyrosine
C propranolol is particularly useful if there is heart failure
D the preoperative finding of a paralysed vocal cord is a contra-indication to surgery
E radioactive iodine has been shown to be followed by an increased incidence of leukaemia

782
Exophthalmos
A may precede the development of frank thyrotoxicosis
B may be aggravated if hypothyroidism is allowed to develop after treatment of thyrotoxicosis
C may cause diplopia which is often first detected when the patient looks upwards and outwards
D can result in loss of visual acuity
E in no circumstances requires surgery, except for lateral tarsorrhaphy

783
In a case of primary hypothyroidism
A the patient may complain of tingling of the fingers even in the absence of anaemia
B the patient is nearly always aware that something is wrong before her doctor is
C frank psychosis is a recognised feature
D tendon reflexes are depressed or absent
E an elevated plasma TSH level is always found

784
In cretinism
A mental impairment is usually reversible even though there has been delay in treatment
B poor feeding will not be observed until the tongue becomes enlarged
C constipation is an early feature
D the appearance of ossification centres in the wrist and heel is delayed relative to chronological age
E parental consanguinity may be causally related to the condition

785
The following statements about goitre are correct:
A Marked elevation of the ESR favours a diagnosis of thyroid carcinoma
B The coincidental presence of nerve deafness in a young patient suggests dyshormonogenesis
C Hashimoto's thyroiditis should rarely be diagnosed in the absence of thyroid antibodies in the serum
D Subacute (de Quervain's) thyroiditis is the most likely cause if hypothyroidism is present
E Concomitant attacks of flushing and diarrhoea raise the possibility of a medullary carcinoma

786
Factors which have been incriminated in the causation of simple goitre include
A excess calcium in drinking water
B viral infection
C prolonged treatment with sulphonamides
D persistent self-medication with some proprietary 'asthma cures'
E a Mendelian recessive gene

787
The concentration of ionised calcium in the plasma
A is lowered after the injection of calcitonin
B is low in patients with hypoalbuminaemia
C is usually low in patients who repeatedly vomit acid gastric juice
D is in part controlled by the action of the parathyroid glands on bone
E is raised in some forms of malignant disease

788
Secondary hyperparathyroidism
A is a recognised cause of calcification of the basal ganglia
B may cause osteomalacia
C may occur as a sequel of chronic renal failure
D only results in osteitis fibrosa if a parathyroid carcinoma is present
E implies autonomous function in parathyroid adenomas

789
Primary hyperparathyroidism
A can often be diagnosed by physical examination
B may present as acute pancreatitis
C may result in renal failure
D may cause thirst and polyuria
E can be excluded if the plasma calcium concentration is normal

790
Hypoparathyroidism
A occurring after partial thyroidectomy is usually permanent
B in an infant may be associated with thymic aplasia
C if idiopathic, may occur at any age
D may be familial
E can usually be adequately controlled by regular oral treatment with parathyroid hormone

791
In the control of tetany
A intravenous isotonic saline is useful if there has been persistent vomiting
B ammonium chloride should not be given to a patient previously overtreated with alkalis
C inhalation of 5 per cent carbon dioxide is helpful if hyperventilation is hysterical
D intravenous calcium gluconate is only helpful if the tetany is due to hypoparathyroidism
E treatment with magnesium may be required if giving calcium fails

792
The following statements about the physiology of the adrenal glands are correct:
A Hyperglycaemia increases the rate of cortisol secretion
B The plasma cortisol level in an unstressed subject is higher at 9 a.m. than at midnight
C Glucocorticoids are antagonistic to insulin
D Aldosterone, weight for weight, has less mineralocorticoid activity than cortisol
E The adrenal cortex synthesises oestrogen in the female only

793
Primary aldosteronism is more likely than secondary aldosteronism to cause
A arterial hypertension
B oedema
C hypokalaemia
D polyuria
E episodic muscular weakness

794
A clue to the aetiology of Addison's disease is given by the presence of
A menorrhagia
B loss of pubic and axillary hair
C calcification in the upper abdomen on plain X-ray
D pigmentation of the buccal mucosa
E diabetes mellitus

795
Addison's disease is more likely than secondary adrenal insufficiency to give rise to
A pigmentation of the buccal mucosa
B loss of body hair
C low blood pressure
D abdominal pain in a crisis
E loss of weight

796
Congenital adrenal insufficiency
A is due to hydroxylase deficiency
B results in the production of large quantities of androgenic steroids
C is easier to diagnose in a male child
D causes premature cessation of growth because of early fusion of the epiphyses
E reduces libido

797
Adrenal insufficiency
A is very unlikely to be present if the serum sodium and potassium concentrations are normal
B is virtually ruled out if hypoglycaemia is absent
C if secondary causes alterations in the diurnal rhythm of cortisol secretion
D is likely to be primary if there is little or no rise in plasma cortisol level after the administration of tetracosactrin depot
E cannot usefully be investigated by the metyrapone test if the patient is taking exogenous corticosteroids in any form

798
Insulin-induced hypoglycaemia
A is the preferred first test if primary adrenocortical insufficiency is suspected
B measures the function of the whole of the hypothalamic-pituitary-adrenal axis
C should be undertaken with caution if hypopituitarism is suspected
D is contra-indicated in an epileptic patient
E should be abandoned as soon as the patient starts to sweat

799
In the treatment of adrenocortical insufficiency
A cortisol is the drug of choice for glucocorticoid replacement
B fludrocortisone is not usually necessary in the secondary variety
C the patient should in no circumstances increase his dose of cortisol without first seeking medical advice
D morphine should be avoided if there is postoperative pain
E hydrocortisone hemisuccinate need only be given intravenously in a crisis if peripheral circulatory failure is present

800
Oral corticosteroids in pharmacological doses are more likely than ACTH to
A inhibit growth in children
B cause peptic ulceration
C produce pigmentation
D result in moonface
E give rise to acne

801
Hypogonadism in the male
A implies failure of the interstitial (Leydig) cells of the testis without any impairment of spermatogenesis
B due to androgen deficiency will respond to oral fluoxymesterone
C results in stunting of growth if it occurs before puberty
D may be due to an XXY sex chromosomal pattern
E may follow venereal disease

802
If the testes in a case of cryptorchidism are present in the inguinal canals
A secondary sex characters fail to develop
B there is an increased risk of testicular carcinoma
C they are more liable to trauma than if they are in the scrotum
D there is a high expectation of sterility if the condition is bilateral
E treatment with chorionic gonadotrophin may be beneficial

803
Impotence
A is usually due to organic disease
B is a recognised early symptom of multiple sclerosis
C is a clear indication for testicular biopsy
D may be complained of by patients with hypopituitarism after replacement treatment with thyroxine and cortisol
E is often cured by the treatment of a varicocele

804
Diabetes mellitus
A affects about 1 per cent of the population in Britain
B is principally a disease of the middle aged and elderly
C may be due to an auto-immune process irrespective of the age of onset of the disease
D is a hereditary disease with a clear dominant form of inheritance in those who become diabetic before the age of 40
E is more likely to occur in women if they are multiparous

805
Biochemical abnormalities which may occur in diabetes mellitus include
A a reduced rate of removal of glucose from the blood by the peripheral tissues
B a circulating insulin antagonist
C decreased glycogenolysis
D increased urinary excretion of magnesium
E depletion of extracellular fluid

806
In diabetes mellitus
A increased osmolality of the glomerular filtrate leads to thirst
B severe depletion of water and electrolytes is more likely to occur in mentally confused patients
C the extent to which increased lipolysis occurs is largely independent of the degree of insulin deficiency
D ketone bodies accumulate because their utilisation by the peripheral tissues is markedly reduced in the absence of insulin
E hyperpnoea occurs when the pH of the blood falls

807
Pathological features of diabetes mellitus include
A marked degeneration of islet cell tissue in diabetes under the age of 40
B evidence of excessive activity of residual beta cells in the elderly
C hyalinisation and fibrosis in the pericapillary space in the islet tissue in the elderly
D reduced permeability of the thickened basement membrane of capillaries
E microangiopathy in the kidney and nervous system as well as in the retina

808
A person with a normal glucose tolerance test is said to be a potential diabetic if
A he is the child of two diabetic parents
B he is overweight
C he develops an abnormal glucose tolerance curve when under severe stress
D he has an identical twin who is diabetic
E he has glycosuria

809
Diabetes mellitus may present with
A epigastric pain and vomiting
B paraesthesiae in the legs
C a change in refraction in the direction of myopia
D vulvitis
E impotence

810
The following statements about glycosuria are correct:
A Clinistix is a glucose-specific test
B Glycosuria is more likely to be discovered by chance in late-onset than in juvenile diabetes
C More of the milder cases of diabetes will be recognised if a sample collected two hours after a meal is tested rather than an overnight specimen of urine
D A 'lag storage' response to a meal (alimentary glycosuria) carries an increased risk of the subsequent development of diabetes
E Glycosuria may result from head injury

811
An oral glucose tolerance test
A cannot be classified as diabetic if no glycosuria is found during the test
B may be normal in a diabetic who also has a phaeochromocytoma
C should be preceded by a restricted carbohydrate diet for three days
D is the most reliable method of making a diagnosis of diabetes mellitus
E may be misleading if performed shortly after a myocardial infarction

812
In the management of diabetes mellitus
A the patient should be warned that he cannot hope to avoid the complication of atherosclerosis however strictly he diets
B the main purpose of a diet is to ensure a flat profile of glycaemia throughout the day
C the daily intake of carbohydrate should be at least 100 g per day in order to avoid ketonuria
D the protein intake should be restricted because amino-acids depress the activity of the beta cells of the pancreas
E the intake of fat should be restricted only if the patient is obese

813
In the treatment of diabetes by oral hypoglycaemic agents
A success cannot be expected in juvenile-onset diabetes
B chlorpropamide may give rise to jaundice
C sulphonylureas are of greatest value in obese patients
D metformin is less likely to cause gastrointestinal side effects than phenformin
E sulphonylureas and biguanides should not be used in combination

814
When insulin is used in the control of diabetes mellitus
A soluble insulin is essential for the treatment of nearly all young patients
B protamine zinc insulin (PZI) is especially useful since it can be given in the same syringe mixed with soluble insulin
C insulin zinc suspension (IZS) crystalline (ultra lente) begins to act at about the same time as PZI
D Isophane (NPH) insulin acts for a much shorter time than globin insulin
E transitory osmotic disturbances in the eye may cause blurring of vision

815
A diabetic patient
A if he is over 40, can expect to control his disease by diet alone
B should be made to experience an insulin reaction if insulin is required to control his disease
C must be instructed in pedicure
D should be advised to test his urine daily at the same time
E may develop a fall in renal threshold during pregnancy

816
Symptoms of hypoglycaemia
A may appear with a blood glucose level of 6.6 mmol/l if the patient is constantly hyperglycaemic
B include mental confusion
C may mimic drunkenness
D come on rapidly irrespective of the type of insulin being used
E are more likely to occur in patients on chlorpropamide than in those on metformin

817
In diabetic ketoacidosis
A the deficit of total body water even in a severe case will not exceed 2 litres
B total body losses of electrolytes can be gauged accurately from serum estimations of sodium and potassium
C abdominal pain and vomiting suggest the presence of acute pancreatitis
D leucocytosis is a characteristic finding
E a life-threatening acidosis may be present even when the blood glucose is as low as 19.4 mmol/l (350mg/100ml)

818
When treating diabetic ketoacidosis
A insulin should be given intravenously as long as there is evidence of peripheral circulatory failure
B the deficit of extracellular fluid should be made good by the infusion of saline isotonic with plasma (0.9 per cent NaCl)
C potassium supplements should not be given until the blood glucose is normal
D gastric aspiration should be undertaken in stuporous patients
E once ketosis has been overcome and the urine is free of sugar, there is no longer any need to give insulin before each oral feed

819
In a diabetic patient who has gone into coma, hypoglycaemic coma is more likely than ketotic coma if there is
A dryness of skin and tongue
B low blood pressure
C a bilateral extensor plantar response
D abdominal pain
E a full pulse

820
The following statements about diabetic complications are correct:
A Gangrene is more likely to occur if peripheral neuropathy is present as well as arterial disease
B The progress of nephropathy can be modified by a high fluid intake
C Photocoagulation is only effective in destroying neovascularisation growing towards the vitreous
D Overflow incontinence of urine due to autonomic neuropathy is best treated by repeated catheterisation
E Peripheral neuropathy improves under treatment with vitamin B1

821
In diabetes mellitus
A cataract only occurs in elderly patients
B there is a predisposition to hydramnios in late pregnancy
C the danger of ketosis in a patient undergoing surgery demands an increased dose of insulin immediately before operation
D the incidence of complications is mainly related to the duration of the disease
E there is a 1:8 chance of a child becoming diabetic if one parent has the disease

822
A pregnant diabetic
A should usually be allowed to proceed to a full term normal delivery
B is very likely to have a baby which is smaller than expected from its gestational age
C will need less insulin as the pregnancy proceeds
D should not be treated with oral hypoglycaemic agents
E may excrete reducing substances other than glucose in the urine

823
Recognised features of Fredrickson's type IIa hyperlipidaemia include
A a clear serum
B hyperuricaemia
C tendon xanthomas
D a high incidence of ischaemic heart disease
E a consistently good response to treatment with a low fat diet

CHAPTER TWELVE

824
In the formation of blood cells
A the liver and spleen normally remain active for about five months after birth
B the medullary cavities are inactive until after birth
C in adults red marrow extends into the shafts of long bones if there is increased demand
D the late normoblast precedes the proerythroblast in the development of red cells
E some lymphocytes are derived from mesenchymal stem cells in the marrow

825
Mature erythrocytes
A are circular biconcave discs
B show a faintly bluish colour with a Romanowsky stain
C derive energy from glucose for electrolyte exchange
D contain the blood group characters in their cytoplasm
E are produced in increased quantities in some forms of renal disease

826
Haemoglobin
A is important in the buffering of carbonic acid
B contains a red pigment which includes ferrous iron
C A contains two alpha and two beta polypeptide chains
D F is normally present in the blood up to the age of about 5 years
E A2 is present only in thalassaemia

827
Iron
A is absorbed in the lower small intestine
B is present in cytochrome
C content of the body is about 5g in an adult
D is conserved by the body so that, in males, the daily loss is only about 1 mg
E is stored in the liver exclusively in the form of ferritin

828
Mature neutrophil granulocytes
A have kidney-shaped nuclei
B have granules containing histamine
C are actively phagocytic to infective organisms
D appear in increased numbers in the peripheral blood in response to emotional stress
E are accompanied by metamyelocytes in the peripheral blood when a severe pyogenic infection is present

829
The following statements are correct:
A Destruction of all formed elements of the blood takes place in cells of the reticuloendothelial system
B Platelets live longer than red cells
C Red cells become broken down as a result of increased enzyme activity weakening their membranes
D The half-life of a red cell, as measured by the radio-active chromium technique, appears to be about 30 days
E Iron liberated from broken-down red cells cannot be re-utilised by the marrow for haemoglobin synthesis

830
In the morphology of red cells
A hypochromia is the characteristic feature of iron deficiency anaemia
B minor degrees of elliptocytosis are of no pathological significance
C polychromasia indicates active production of new red cells
D punctate basophilia occurs only in chronic lead poisoning
E normoblasts may be present in the peripheral blood in leukaemia

831
The following statements about white blood cells are correct:
A Infants commonly respond to infections by producing a lymphocytosis
B Leucopenia is a good prognostic sign in severe pyogenic infections
C Eosinophilia is found in advancing tuberculosis
D Monocytosis is a recognised finding in malaria
E Myelocytes appear in the peripheral blood in adult patients with myelofibrosis

832
In iron deficiency anaemia
A the tongue is heavily furred
B brittleness of the nails precedes the concavity of koilonychia
C objective signs of disease of the central nervous system are never found unless some other disease is also present
D the haemoglobin may fall as low as 7 g/dl before symptoms appear
E the bone marrow may show a megaloblastic reaction in very severe cases

833
When oral iron is prescribed for a patient with iron deficiency anaemia
A it should be given before meals in order to increase its absorption
B ferrous sulphate is the cheapest preparation
C it is advisable to keep him in bed if the haemoglobin is below 4g/dl
D folic acid should be prescribed in addition if the haemoglobin is less than 8g/dl
E very little will be absorbed once the haemoglobin has been restored to normal

834
Megaloblasts in the bone marrow
A have a more loosely woven chromatin network in the nucleus than normoblasts
B are best distinguished from normoblasts by their deeply basophilic cytoplasm
C may appear as a result of dietary deficiency
D may appear as a complication of jejunal diverticulosis
E in Britain most often appear as a result of gastric surgery

835
Addisonian pernicious anaemia
A is rare before the age of 30
B only rarely occurs in relatives of an affected patient
C may well have an auto-immune basis
D may be present even if there are some normoblasts in the bone marrow
E is accompanied by hyperbilirubinaemia

836
In Addisonian pernicious anaemia
A weight loss is a common feature
B achlorhydria is always present
C dementia is a recognised complication
D thrombocytosis is characteristic
E the absorption from the alimentary tract of cyanocobalamin labelled with radioactive cobalt is impaired

837
In the treatment of Addisonian pernicious anaemia
A blood transfusion is obligatory if the haemoglobin is less than 7g/dl
B the reticulocyte count reaches a maximum about six days after treatment is commenced
C the bone marrow does not revert to a normoblastic state until one month after the first injection of hydroxocobalamin
D if there are objective signs of subacute combined degeneration of the cord, hydroxocobalamin should be given cautiously and in a reduced dose
E large doses of oral vitamin B12 prove satisfactory in place of monthly injections after the first year of therapy

838
Folate deficiency occurs
A rarely in Britain as a result of dietary deficiency except in the elderly
B as a result of anticonvulsant therapy
C in pregnancy only if there is associated vitamin B12 deficiency
D equally commonly in infants in Britain and in developing countries
E in leukaemia

839
Pancytopenia
A follows thyroxine deficiency
B if idiopathic, is usually fatal in about six months
C may follow treatment with indomethacin
D due to drugs may develop months after the cessation of treatment
E may respond to treatment with oxymetholone

840
Recognised consequences of excessive blood destruction include
A bilirubinuria
B reduction of plasma haptoglobins
C reticulocytosis
D haemoglobinuria
E spherocytosis

841
In hereditary spherocytosis
A symptoms usually appear in childhood
B crises may be associated with rigors
C the bone marrow shows normoblastic hyperplasia
D haemolytic transfusion reactions are uncommon
E the Coombs' test is typically positive

842
Haemolytic anaemia which occurs
A as a result of infection with streptococci is common in Britain
B in malignant disease may depend on autoimmune factors
C in a patient with chronic leukaemia is more likely to be due to treatment than to the disease itself
D in association with viral pneumonia is likely to be due to a cold-antibody reaction
E as a result of transfusion with incompatible blood should be treated with hydrocortisone

843
Haemolytic disease of the newborn
A can be prevented in future pregnancies by giving the Rh negative mother of an Rh positive child anti D immunoglobulin within 72 hours of the child's birth
B tends to increase in severity in successive pregnancies
C is to be expected in every subsequent child born to a Rh negative mother who has had one Rh positive baby
D causes deep jaundice which is immediately apparent as soon as the child is born
E should always be treated by exchange transfusion once it has occurred

844
In a case of auto-immune (acquired) haemolytic anaemia
A there is usually a history of transfusion with incompatible blood
B the prognosis is more serious than in hereditary haemolytic anaemia
C a positive Coombs' test provides absolute diagnostic proof
D the fragility of the red cells is decreased
E splenectomy should be carried out if corticosteroid treatment fails

845
Recognised features of an incompatible blood transfusion include
A fever
B oliguria
C an onset only after about 500ml or more have been transfused
D bradycardia
E praecordial pain

846
An increase in the number of circulating red cells
A is found in association with extensive burns
B is a recognised complication of hepatoma
C is usually accompanied by leucocytosis and thrombocytosis in patients with chronic pulmonary disease
D if due to polycythaemia vera, is usually accompanied by a low leucocyte alkaline phosphatase score
E should be treated with ^{32}P or busulphan if the PaO_2 is low

847
In a patient with agranulocytosis
A there is usually no discoverable cause
B if imipramine is being taken it should be stopped
C the prognosis is worse if the condition is chronic
D treatment with antibiotics and blood transfusion may be life-saving
E the bone marrow usually shows many early myelocytes

848
Patients suffering from infectious mononucleosis
A are usually middle aged
B develop antibodies to the Epstein-Barr virus in the serum during recovery
C are often profoundly anaemic
D are much more likely to develop a rash if ampicillin is used in treatment
E have clinical and haematological features similar to those of toxoplasmosis

849
Acute lymphoblastic leukaemia
A is the commonest lethal malignant disease in childhood
B unlike chronic leukaemias, does not occur in a subleukaemic form
C may be confused with infectious mononucleosis in the early stage of the disease
D causes a bleeding tendency which can be reduced by treatment with prednisolone
E responds less well to antimitotic agents than acute myeloblastic leukaemia

850
In chronic myeloid leukaemia
A attacks of left upper abdominal pain may be due to splenic infarction
B the spleen is larger than in other forms of leukaemia
C it is important to reduce the white cell count as quickly as possible so as to minimise the risk of uric acid nephropathy
D the presence of an extra chromosome 22 (trisomy 22) is characteristic
E an increasing number of myeloblasts in the peripheral blood is a bad prognostic sign

851
Chronic lymphatic leukaemia
A occurs in a younger age group than chronic myeloid leukaemia
B only causes anaemia late on in its course
C gives rise to an increased tendency to develop infections
D should be treated vigorously in its early stages even in the absence of serious symptoms
E is often associated with a positive Paul Bunnell test

852
Lymphadenoma (Hodgkin's disease)
A characteristically gives rise to enlarged painful lymph nodes
B is characterised by lymphocytosis in the peripheral blood
C causes troublesome pruritus in about 10 per cent of cases
D should be treated with chemotherapy when the disease is advanced
E carries a prognosis which bears little or no relation to the histological appearance of the lymph nodes

853
Enlargement of the spleen *and* lymph nodes is a characteristic feature of
A reticulum-cell sarcoma
B chronic myeloid leukaemia
C infectious mononucleosis
D hypersplenism
E chronic lymphatic leukaemia

854
The following substances are normally present in the circulating blood:
A thromboplastin
B plasminogen
C Christmas factor
D fibrin
E antihaemophilic factor

855
The following haemorrhagic disorders are due to a defect in the clotting mechanism:
A senile purpura
B Henoch-Schönlein purpura
C haemophilia
D scurvy
E hereditary haemorrhagic telangiectasia

856
Idiopathic thrombocytopenic purpura
A is exceptional under the age of 40
B is usually associated with a palpable
   spleen
C is accompanied by a bleeding time
   which may be prolonged to 15 minutes
D shows haematological improvement
   within a few minutes of splenectomy
E is not usually influenced by treatment
   with corticosteroids

857
**The following statements about
haemophilia are correct:**
A The abnormal gene is carried on one of
   the X chromosomes
B The thromboplastin generation test may
   be abnormal even if the coagulation
   time is normal
C Cryoprecipitate is the most widely used
   form of treatment
D Haematomas should be treated by
   aspiration
E Female relations of a haemophilic male
   should be strongly advised not to have
   children

CHAPTER THIRTEEN

858
Rheumatoid arthritis
A most commonly arises before the age
   of 30
B affects males more often than females
C may be precipitated by emotional
   disturbances
D is characterised in its early stages by
   swelling and congestion of the synovial
   membrane and overlying connective
   tissue
E in its later stages is typically associated
   with progressive destruction of the
   articular cartilage

859
**Recognised features of rheumatoid
arthritis include**
A hyperplastic lymph nodes
B osteoarthrosis in the later stages
C granulomatous lesions of the sclera
D an acute febrile onset
E early involvement of the sacroiliac
   joints

860
In rheumatoid arthritis
A the characteristic deformity in the
   hands is anterior subluxation of the
   metacarpophalangeal joints and ulnar
   deviation of the fingers
B the subcutaneous nodules contain
   giant cells and numerous plasma cells
C the most common site for
   subcutaneous nodules is over the
   terminal interphalangeal joint
D amyloidosis is a recognised late
   complication
E diffuse vasculitis is a common feature

861
**Recognised extra-articular
manifestations of rheumatoid arthritis
include**
A leg ulcers
B pneumoconiosis
C pericarditis
D pleural effusion
E peripheral neuropathy

862
Characteristic features of active rheumatoid arthritis include
A fever
B macrocytic anaemia
C leucopenia
D hypoalbuminaemia
E positive latex fixation test

863
The following statements are correct:
A The joint pain is of a flitting character in rheumatic fever
B In gonococcal arthritis the organism can be seen on direct smear or isolated on culture of synovial fluid in the majority of cases
C Fibrous ankylosis is the usual end-result in joints involved by Reiter's disease
D The Rose-Waaler test is negative in psoriatic arthritis
E Acute pyogenic arthritis is a recognised complication of rheumatoid arthritis

864
In the acute phase of rheumatoid arthritis
A the patient should be confined to bed
B foot and quadriceps exercises should be performed daily by all patients confined to bed
C a high protein diet is indicated
D vitamin supplements are important adjuncts to therapy in all patients
E painful joints should be immobilised in skin tight plaster of Paris splints

865
The following statements regarding the treatment of rheumatoid arthritis are correct:
A Aspirin is the most valuable anti-inflammatory agent available for the control of symptoms
B Codeine phosphate acts by inhibiting prostaglandin biosynthesis
C Paracetamol should be given in a dose of 1 gm/day
D Phenylbutazone should only be used when the response to aspirin has been unsatisfactory
E Propionic acid derivatives are employed because they are free from gastro-intestinal side effects

866
Recognised side effects of phenylbutazone include
A oedema
B haematemesis
C agranulocytosis
D alopecia
E chromosomal abnormalities

867
Regarding corticosteroid usage in rheumatoid arthritis
A the optimum dosage of prednisolone for maintenance therapy is 15 mg daily
B taking prednisolone with food will reduce the incidence of peptic ulceration
C it is usually possible to discontinue prednisolone after a few years of treatment
D intra-articular injections of hydrocortisone acetate will reduce joint pain and swelling
E hydrocortisone eye drops (1.5 per cent solution) are of value in the treatment of inflammatory complications in the eye

868
In the treatment of rheumatoid arthritis
A ACTH is significantly less effective than oral prednisolone
B tetracosactrin has caused fatal anaphylactic reactions
C gold salts are of unproven value
D dermatitis is the most common adverse reaction to gold salts
E bone marrow depression is a recognised complication of gold therapy

869
The following statements are correct:
A Dimercaprol stimulates the hepatic detoxification of gold salts
B Patients treated with long-term chloroquine should have full ophthalmic assessment every 3-6 months
C Oral iron will correct the anaemia of rheumatoid arthritis in most cases
D Tendon rupture is a recognised complication of rheumatoid disease
E Synovectomy may be followed by local remission of activity for prolonged periods

870
In juvenile rheumatoid arthritis (Still's disease)
A the spleen is often enlarged
B leucopenia is more common than leucocytosis
C the Rose-Waaler test is positive in the majority of patients
D growth is not retarded unless prednisolone is used in treatment
E the cervical spine is often involved

871
In Sjögren's syndrome
A dryness of the mouth is characteristic
B keratoconjunctivitis sicca is due to atrophy of the tear ducts
C recurrent respiratory infection is a recognised complication
D hair loss is a recognised feature
E the test for rheumatoid factor is negative in the majority of cases

872
Ankylosing spondylitis
A is commonest after the age of 40
B affects males more often than females
C is characteristically associated with a positive test for rheumatoid factor
D is associated with the histocompatibility antigen HLA-B27 in more than 90 per cent of cases
E typically involves the sacro-iliac joints at an early stage

873
In ankylosing spondylitis
A the onset is typically acute
B repeated attacks of backache are a recognised presenting feature
C early morning pain and stiffness are characteristic features
D sciatic pain is a common feature
E the hip joints are characteristically spared

874
Recognised associations with ankylosing spondylitis include
A iritis
B aortic regurgitation
C ulcerative colitis
D kyphosis
E urethritis

875
In the treatment of ankylosing spondylitis
A corticosteroids are without effect
B immobilisatiion in the active stage should be of very limited duration
C radiotherapy can produce apparent arrest of the disease
D phenylbutazone is particularly effective
E physiotherapy has little effect

876
Characteristic features of systemic lupus erythematosus include.
A Raynaud's phenomenon
B pleural effusion
C erosive arthritis of the rheumatoid type
D alopecia
E exacerbation following exposure to sunlight

877
Systemic lupus erythematosus
A may be induced by the administration of sulphonamides
B is equally common in men and women
C characteristically causes a rash of butterfly distribution on the face
D usually causes leucocytosis
E is a recognised cause of renal failure

878
In systemic lupus erythematosus
A antinuclear factor (ANF) is present in the majority of cases
B the titre of anti-DNA antibodies correlates well with the activity of the disease
C serum complement levels are characteristically raised
D high dosage of prednisolone is indicated if acute manifestations are present
E chloroquine is valuable in reversing the renal lesions

879
Dermatomyositis
A is characteristically associated with a positive LE cell phenomenon
B is characterised by focal or segmental necrosis of voluntary muscles
C in the acute form is more common in adults than in children
D is typically associated with a raised serum creatine kinase
E in the chronic form has a recognised association with malignant disease

880
Polymyalgia rheumatica
A affects elderly women more than men
B has a recognised association with cranial arteritis
C is characterised by pain in the calves
D is typically associated with fever and weight loss
E should be treated with azathioprine or cyclophosphamide

881
Gout
A of the primary variety results from an inborn error of purine metabolism
B typically presents with multiple peripheral joint involvement
C has a recognised association with polycythaemia
D is the most likely diagnosis when a young woman presents with acute inflammation of a single joint
E of the secondary variety may be precipitated by treatment with frusemide

882
The following statements about gout are correct:
A An acute attack may be precipitated by a surgical operation
B A family history is obtained in only 25 per cent of those with the primary variety
C There is deposition of urates in the kidneys
D Cyst-like areas found in radiographs of affected joints are due to urate deposits
E The ESR is typically normal in acute attacks

883
In the treatment of gout
A indomethacin is the drug of choice in acute cases
B probenecid increases the urinary excretion of uric acid
C allopurinol increases the urinary excretion of xanthine
D dietary restrictions are of primary importance in all patients
E allopurinol is contra-indicated if renal function is impaired

884
Osteoarthrosis
A is characterised by degeneration of the articular cartilage and the formation of bony outgrowths
B is a recognised sequel of malalignment following a fracture
C predominates in the weight-bearing joints
D typically leads to bony ankylosis
E is associated with muscular wasting in a minority of cases

885
The following statements are correct:
A Osteomyelitis seldom occurs before the age of 12
B *Staph. pyogenes* is the most common organism involved in osteomyelitis
C Osteomyelitis typically presents with local pain and systemic upset
D Penicillin is the most effective treatment for acute staphylococcal osteomyelitis
E Tuberculosis mainly affects the posterior parts of the vertebral bodies

886
Paget's disease (osteitis deformans)
A is seldom seen before the age of 50
B is a recognised cause of deafness
C is characterised by decreased osteoblastic activity
D is characteristically associated with hypercalcaemia
E may be complicated by spontaneous fractures which heal slowly if at all

CHAPTER FOURTEEN

887
In the diagnosis of neurological disease, the following general principles apply:
A Vascular disturbances develop rapidly but less acutely than inflammatory lesions
B Very rapid deterioration excludes a cerebral tumour
C The history is more important than the physical examination in the determination of the pathological process involved
D The disabilities caused by degenerative disorders and tumours usually have a similar time course
E A remittent history is typical of motor neurone disease

888
An upper motor neurone lesion associated with
A epilepsy is probably in the internal capsule
B dysphasia is probably in the cortex
C hemianopia is probably in the internal capsule
D a contralateral cranial nerve lesion is probably in the brain stem
E segmental sensory disturbance is probably in the spinal cord

889
Characteristic features of a lower motor neurone lesion include
A loss of muscle tone
B muscular wasting
C clonus
D abnormal electrical excitability of the affected muscles
E contracture of muscles

890
The following statements are correct:
A The synthesis of sensory information is mainly carried out in the non-dominant parietal lobe
B Lesions of the thalamus may cause severe pain
C Lesions in the cortex do not abolish any forms of sensation
D Lesions in the supramarginal and angular gyri of the dominant hemisphere cause receptive dysphasia
E Perceptual rivalry can be elicited by stimulating the two sides of the body in turn

891
The segmental levels of the common tendon reflexes are as follows:
A supinator : C 5-6
B biceps : C 5-6
C triceps : C 7
D knee : L 1-2
E ankle : S 4-5

892
The following statements about neurological disorders of the bladder are correct:
A A lesion of the upper sacral segments of the cord can cause retention of urine
B A lesion in the cord above the sacral segments causes either incontinence or retention
C Stimulation of parasympathetic fibres in the pelvic nerves causes emptying of the bladder
D The bladder may shrink as a result of a lesion in the thoracic segments of the cord
E A lesion of the pudendal nerves leads to automatic bladder emptying

893
The following signs are suggestive of damage to the prefrontal lobe of the cerebral cortex:
A positive grasp reflex
B astereognosis
C loss of appreciation by the patient of the consequences of his actions
D olfactory hallucinations
E receptive dysphasia

894
Recognised causes of papilloedema include
A cranial arteritis
B cavernous sinus thrombosis
C severe respiratory failure
D thrombosis of the central retinal vein
E migraine

895
A woman of 40 complains of continuous diplopia during the past month. Examination shows drooping of the right eyelid which she is unable to overcome by maximum voluntary effort. The right eye is deviated to the right and diplopia occurs in all directions of gaze, except maximum deviation to the right. The left eye is normal. These findings might be due to
A raised intracranial pressure from any cause
B diabetes mellitus
C multiple sclerosis
D meningovascular syphilis
E a lesion of the cervical sympathetic chain

896
The pain of trigeminal neuralgia
A is characteristically first felt in the area supplied by the ophthalmic division of the trigeminal nerve
B may provoke spasm of the facial muscles
C characteristically persists for several hours at a time
D may be precipitated by touching the face
E is commoner in elderly patients than in the young

897
In Bell's palsy
A the ability to wrinkle the forehead on the affected side is preserved
B there is ipsilateral loss of taste sensation from the posterior third of the tongue
C the eye on the affected side cannot be closed
D sensation from the skin of the face is not affected
E if commencing recovery is seen within one week from the onset a good prognosis may be given

898
Recognised causes of vertigo include
A atheroma of the basilar artery
B vestibular neuronitis
C medication with quinine
D head injury
E petit mal

899
In Ménière's syndrome
A there is nearly always progressive nerve deafness
B the vertigo is usually of sudden onset
C attacks may be accompanied by nausea and vomiting
D tinnitus is a late manifestation
E the usual cause is an acoustic neuroma

900
A man of 60 is found to have wasting of the right side of the tongue. When protruded the tongue deviates to the right. The cause might be
A a lesion of the internal capsule
B carcinoma of the naso-pharynx
C Paget's disease
D myasthenia gravis
E pseudobulbar palsy

901
The following are components of Horner's syndrome:
A ptosis
B constriction of the pupil
C excessive sweating over the face
D enophthalmos
E paralysis of accommodation

902
Characteristic features of Friedreich's ataxia include
A absent ankle reflexes
B extensor plantar responses
C an irregular course punctuated by relapses and remissions
D loss of vibration sense
E pes cavus

903
An upper motor neurone lesion is a recognised feature of
A subacute combined degeneration of the cord
B hepato-lenticular degeneration (Wilson's disease)
C amyotrophic lateral sclerosis
D Bell's palsy
E facio-scapulo-humeral muscular dystrophy

904
Temporal lobe epilepsy may give rise to
A hallucinations of smell
B the 'déjà vu' phenomenon
C disturbance of consciousness
D antisocial acts
E paralysis of one or more limbs for an hour or two after the attack

905
A man of 60 has been well until two months ago when he had the first of seven typical grand mal attacks. Among other possible causes you should consider
A alcoholism
B neurosyphilis
C hypoglycaemia
D hepato-lenticular degeneration (Wilson's disease)
E cerebrovascular disease

906
If phenobarbitone medication failed to control grand mal epilepsy it would be worth trying
A phenytoin
B methylphenidate hydrochloride
C primidone
D clonidine
E carbamazepine

907
The following drugs are of value in the treatment of petit mal:
A amphetamine sulphate
B ethosuximide
C phenobarbitone
D imipramine
E sodium valproate

908
Complications of the long-term treatment of grand mal epilepsy include
A drowsiness
B hypochromic anaemia
C osteomalacia
D gum hypertrophy
E ataxia

909
A diagnosis of narcolepsy would be supported by the following findings:
A attacks in which the patient falls to the ground unconscious and rises again immediately
B episodes of paralysis of the limbs without loss of consciousness during the day
C episodes of paralysis on waking or falling asleep
D attacks of sleep during the day from which the patient can be aroused only with difficulty
E terrifying hallucinations as the patient is falling asleep

910
There is a good prospect of long-term survival after surgical removal of
A medulloblastoma
B astrocytoma
C meningioma
D acoustic neuroma
E oligodendroglioma

911
Tumours in the posterior fossa of the skull
A are commoner in childhood than in adult life
B seldom give rise to papilloedema
C sometimes cause paralysis of the sixth cranial nerve
D should not in general be investigated by lumbar puncture
E respond dramatically to cytotoxic drugs such as cyclophosphamide

912
Common sites for the development of meningiomas include
A the sphenoidal ridges
B the cerebellar vermis
C the olfactory grooves
D the spinal cord
E the convexities of the hemispheres

913
Recognised accompaniments of raised intracranial pressure include
A early morning headache
B generalised epilepsy
C vomiting
D tachycardia
E personality changes

914
Papilloedema due to raised intracranial pressure
A is usually discovered because the patient complains of severe loss of visual acuity
B is typically bilateral
C if rapid in development may be accompanied by haemorrhages radiating out from the optic disc
D characteristically causes a central scotoma
E causes pain and tenderness in the affected eye

915
In the investigation of suspected cerebral tumour
A X-ray of the chest may yield important information
B electroencephalography cannot be expected to show more than the diffuse slow waves of raised intracranial pressure
C a reduced sugar content in the cerebrospinal fluid is sometimes found in carcinomatosis of the meninges
D echoencephalography is capable of lateralising a space-occupying lesion
E arteriography is less often needed since the advent of computerised axial tomography

916
The following intracranial structures are sensitive to pain:
A corpus callosum
B sagittal sinus
C internal carotid arteries
D dura at the base of the brain
E dura over the cerebral hemispheres

917
Migraine
A tends to run in families
B usually starts in early childhood
C should not be diagnosed unless the pain is confined to one side of the head
D may cause paraesthesiae or weakness of one half of the body
E may be precipitated by eating certain foods

918
The visual symptoms of migraine
A usually develop about twenty minutes after the onset of the headache
B may include temporary defects in the visual fields
C are due to dilatation of cortical arteries
D include photophobia
E seldom last longer than half an hour

919
There is a high risk of cerebral embolism in a patient suffering from
A atrial fibrillation
B myocardial infarction
C left atrial myxoma
D deep vein thrombosis in the calf
E infective endocarditis

920
Management of the hemiplegic patient should include
A maintenance of fluid and calorie (kilojoule) intake by the intravenous route only
B a short course of anticoagulant therapy
C very cautious mobilisation
D occupational therapy
E reduction of blood pressure if it remains persistently high

921
The following are recognised modes of presentation of a cerebral aneurysm:
A Sudden onset of severe occipital headache followed by unconsciousness
B Recurring episodes of headache which may be mistaken for migraine
C Pain in the distribution of the ophthalmic division of the trigeminal nerve
D Oculomotor palsies
E Tinnitus and deafness

922
A labourer of 45 is admitted having been found unconscious in his lodging-house. He is totally unresponsive to all stimuli and has marked neck stiffness. Possible diagnoses include
A severe alcoholic intoxication
B subarachnoid haemorrhage
C pyogenic meningitis
D viral meningitis
E barbiturate overdosage

923
The protein concentration in the cerebro-spinal fluid is very high in the presence of
A spinal block
B spinal neurofibroma
C viral meningitis
D Guillain-Barré polyneuropathy
E neurosyphilis

924
A low glucose level in the cerebrospinal fluid is compatible with a diagnosis of
A pyogenic meningitis
B viral meningitis
C tuberculous meningitis
D carcinomatous meningitis
E poliomyelitis

925
A spinal epidural abscess
A is usually painless
B may cause radiological changes in the spine
C is best treated conservatively with antibiotics and physiotherapy
D usually causes a polymorphonuclear leucocytosis in the peripheral blood
E may cause incontinence of urine

926
Intracerebral abscess is a recognised complication of
A bronchiectasis
B otitis media
C frontal sinusitis
D head injury
E infective endocarditis

927
Chronic intracranial abscess
A usually causes fever
B may cause papilloedema
C should not be diagnosed in the absence of a polymorphonuclear leucocytosis in the peripheral blood
D commonly causes characteristic abnormalities in the EEG
E even if successfully treated, is followed by epilepsy in a high proportion of patients

928
Tuberculous meningitis
A is commoner in children than in adults
B progresses more rapidly in children than in adults
C is fatal in a few weeks if untreated
D is a recognised cause of hypertrophic pachymeningitis in the cervical region
E should not be treated with antituberculous chemotherapy until the organism has been isolated

929
Acute lymphocytic choriomeningitis
A is commoner in children than in the elderly
B may be difficult to distinguish from non-paralytic poliomyelitis
C differs from tuberculous meningitis in that, in the early stages of the latter, the predominant cells in the CSF are polymorphonuclear leucocytes
D should be treated energetically with cytarabine
E carries a poor prognosis unless treatment is started before the third day of illness

930
Characteristic features of the Argyll Robertson pupil include
A wide dilatation
B reaction to convergence
C failure to react to light
D atrophy of the iris
E irregularity

931
In the following clinical situations it is important to exclude syphilis as the cause:
A A stroke in a young patient
B The onset of epilepsy in the fifth decade
C Carpal tunnel syndrome occurring in a male patient
D Ataxia which is worse in the dark or on closing the eyes
E A stamping gait

932
The following statements regarding neurosyphilis are correct:
A Almost all patients with tabes dorsalis have a positive Wassermann reaction in the c.s.f.
B Treatment of neurosyphilis should be continued until the c.s.f. WR is negative
C Intramuscular procaine benzylpenicillin is the treatment of choice
D Nearly all patients with active disease show abnormally high cell counts in the c.s.f.
E The raised c.s.f. cell count usually returns to normal as a result of effective therapy

933
Viral encephalitis
A may be caused by any virus capable of causing meningitis
B rarely causes any disturbance of consciousness
C may cause epilepsy
D if due to herpes simplex virus, should be treated with intravenous idoxuridine
E causes the c.s.f. glucose concentration to fall to very low levels

934
In acute anterior poliomyelitis
A the incubation period is about 3 weeks
B mild fever and headache may be the sole clinical manifestations
C there may be signs of meningeal irritation
D there may be c.s.f. changes which are indistinguishable from those of acute lymphocytic choriomeningitis
E muscular paralysis is irreversible

935
In herpes zoster
A the virus responsible is the same as that causing chicken-pox
B the infection is confined to the posterior root ganglia and does not extend to the spinal cord or brain
C the first symptom is pain unaccompanied by any visible change in the skin
D the eruption heals without scarring
E there may be permanent loss of sensation in the area of skin involved

936
The following are recognised consequences of herpes zoster:
A corneal ulceration
B severe and intractable pain, lasting for months or years after healing of the skin lesions
C facial paralysis
D segmental muscle wasting
E neuroma

937
Common features of multiple sclerosis include
A a progressive downhill course without remissions especially if the disease begins in early adult life
B episodes of blindness in one or other eye
C ataxic nystagmus
D intractable pain
E urgency of micturition

938
In multiple sclerosis
A females are more often affected than males
B the prevalence in Britain is lower than in Central Africa
C there is good evidence of a genetic aetiology
D females are more severely affected than males
E the earlier the onset the worse the prognosis

939
Recognised features of parkinsonism include
A hypokinesis
B extensive sensory loss
C rigidity
D dementia
E tremor

940
In a patient presenting with parkinsonism, the following findings would suggest that paralysis agitans was not the correct diagnosis:
A bilateral extensor plantar responses
B a shuffling gait
C slow, monotonous speech
D loss of emotional control
E oculogyric crises

941
The following drugs, given alone, are of value in the treatment of parkinsonism:
A carbidopa
B monoamineoxidase inhibitors
C bromocriptine
D benztropine
E alpha-methyldopa

942
Wilson's disease (hepato-lenticular degeneration)
A is inherited as an autosomal recessive disorder
B is clinically obvious at birth
C is characterised by a high serum caeruloplasmin concentration
D may cause progressive dementia
E can be arrested by the administration of penicillamine by mouth

943
In spinal cord compression
A tuberculosis is more likely to be the cause than tumour in Britain
B urgency of micturition is an early symptom
C pain does not usually occur until motor weakness is obvious
D there may be difficulty in differentiation from multiple sclerosis
E surgical decompression is particularly useful if there is leukaemic infiltration

944
Kernicterus
A is commoner in premature than in full-term babies
B may follow any severe neonatal jaundice
C is less likely to develop in a full-term baby once it has reached the age of 10 days
D produces neurological changes which can be reversed by appropriate therapy
E may result in deafness

945
The movements
A in parkinsonism are slow and lack precision
B of chorea are stereotyped
C of ballism are 'flinging'
D of a person suffering from a tic are unpredictable
E of athetosis are 'writhing'

946
Recognised features of motor neurone disease include
A an insidious onset
B painful cramps in the legs
C muscular wasting
D Argyll Robertson pupils
E raised c.s.f. protein concentration

947
The combination of wasting of the small muscles of the hand and extensor plantar responses is compatible with a diagnosis of
A syringomyelia
B motor neurone disease
C progressive muscular dystrophy
D general paralysis of the insane
E acute infective polyneuritis (Guillain-Barré syndrome)

948
Characteristic findings in cervical spondylosis include
A pain of radicular distribution
B upper motor neurone type weakness in the legs
C sensory loss in the upper limbs
D increased incidence in older patients
E pain and limitation of movement of the neck

949
Sciatica
A is pain in the distribution of the sciatic nerve when it is due to herniation of an intervertebral disc
B is exacerbated by coughing or sneezing
C is almost never accompanied by sensory loss
D may be accompanied by weakness of the calf muscles
E causes increased lumbar lordosis

950
Deficiency of vitamin B_{12} may cause
A paraesthesiae in the extremities
B wasting of the muscles of the tongue
C optic atrophy
D mental impairment
E Argyll Robertson pupils

951
Wernicke's encephalopathy
A is due to pyridoxine deficiency
B commonly causes nystagmus
C may cause loss of pupillary reflexes
D may cause disorders of ocular movement
E is often due to alcoholism

952
The features of Brown-Séquard syndrome include
A loss of temperature sensation in the leg opposite to the lesion
B xanthochromia in the cerebrospinal fluid
C a band of hyperaesthesia at the level of the lesion but on the opposite side
D an extensor plantar response on the side of the lesion
E loss of proprioceptive sense in the leg on the same side as the lesion

953
In a paraplegic patient
A prophylactic antibiotic treatment prevents the formation of urinary calculi
B pressure sores are only likely to occur if there is sensory loss
C it is dangerous to encourage emptying of the bladder by manual compression of the lower abdomen
D the incidence of flexor spasms can be reduced by regular passive movements of the limbs
E faecal impaction is preventable

954
The carpal tunnel syndrome
A typically remits during pregnancy
B is associated with wasting of the lumbrical and interosseous muscles
C may interfere with sleep
D is a recognised complication of thyrotoxicosis
E is rarely bilateral

955
Polyneuropathy due to
A the Guillain-Barré syndrome spares the cranial nerves
B lead poisoning is characterised by extensive sensory loss
C diabetes may be manifest as postural hypotension
D alcohol causes severe pain
E acute intermittent porphyria is often associated with hypertension

956
Non-metastatic neurological complications of carcinoma include
A progressive dementia
B cerebellar ataxia
C carpal tunnel syndrome
D a myasthenic syndrome
E meralgia paraesthetica

957
In a patient complaining of muscular weakness, the following findings are characteristic of myasthenia gravis:
A weakness made worse by vigorous exercise
B diplopia
C weakness predominantly affecting the legs
D improvement after injection of edrophonium
E fluctuating intensity of symptoms

958
The following are characteristic of progressive muscular dystrophy:
A symmetrical wasting and weakness
B widespread fasciculation
C impaired joint position sense
D intact tendon reflexes except in late stages
E severely shortened life-span in all types

959
Dilatation of intracranial or extracranial arteries is thought to be the mechanism responsible for the headache
A of meningitis
B of chronic respiratory failure
C of migraine
D following lumbar puncture
E of post-herpetic neuralgia

960
The following features would favour a diagnosis of psychogenic headache:
A The pain is worst on waking and gets better as the day wears on
B The pain is felt exclusively at the vertex
C The patient appears clinically depressed
D The pain interferes with sleep
E The pain is of a 'pressing' character

961
In intracranial haemorrhage the following signs are indicative of involvement of the site mentioned:
A hemiplegia: internal capsule
B pin-point pupils: pons
C vertigo: thalamus
D sub-hyaloid haemorrhage: cerebellum
E neck rigidity: 3rd ventricle

962
The prognosis in stroke is relatively poor if
A the patient loses consciousness
B the stroke was due to cerebral embolism rather than haemorrhage or infarction
C dementia develops
D hypertension is not controlled
E the patient has defects in conjugate gaze

963
Normal pressure hydrocephalus
A is a recognised cause of dementia
B causes narrowing of the ventricles
C is thought to be initiated by some lesion causing obstruction to the flow of c.s.f.
D has a strongly hereditary incidence
E may be treatable by surgery in some cases

964
The following are recognised manifestations of brain-stem infarction:
A severe headache
B bitemporal hemianopia
C diplopia
D motor dysphasia
E nystagmus

CHAPTER FIFTEEN

965
Psychiatric illness
A is to a very large extent treated by psychiatrists
B rarely occurs in association with physical illness
C can be effectively treated by physical methods
D is often associated with difficulties in interpersonal relationships
E is easier for the doctor to understand if he is sufficiently imaginative to use his own life experience to grasp what the patient is suffering

966
In dealing with a patient suffering from a psychiatric illness
A the doctor must at all costs preserve an attitude of detached authority
B an optimistic therapeutic approach is likely to result in a fuller history
C there is no way in which a paranoid patient can be prevented from thinking that the doctor is part of the plot against him
D a question and answer interviewing technique often constrains the patient
E the patient's first account of his illness is more likely to be relevant than subsequent versions

967
Major psychiatric disorders (psychoses) include
A organic dementia
B sexual deviation
C schizophrenia
D alcoholism
E sociopathy

968
Recognised causes of delirium include
A brain trauma
B ageing
C encephalitis
D multiple sclerosis
E hepatic failure

969
Recognised causes of dementia include
A Sydenham's chorea
B neurosyphilis
C pellagra
D carbon monoxide poisoning
E heart failure

970
Personality disorder
A may be difficult to diagnose in a psychotic patient
B may lead the patient to seek treatment because of his inability to get on with other people
C is not usually associated with other psychiatric illness
D may not be recognised by the patient suffering from it
E is almost never associated with psychosomatic illness such as asthma

971
In the course of a child's development
A an I.Q. of 60 implies that no benefit can be expected from teaching and social training
B if severe mental retardation is established, a definite physical cause is nearly always found
C fear of strangers develops from the age of eight months
D girls do not develop intense affection for their fathers until puberty is reached
E becoming a member of a group does not interfere with successful identity formation

972
The following statements about defence mechanisms are correct:
A Women who remain unaware of their sexual impulses are showing 'denial'
B A sexually deprived woman who believes that neighbours view her as sexually promiscuous illustrates the ill effect of 'projection' in a patient who has previously relied on 'repression'
C A surgeon's matter-of-fact manner is an example of 'reaction formation'
D 'Sublimation' is at work when a schoolmaster interferes sexually with boys
E A son, dominated by his father, who becomes a timid subservient adult is showing 'overcompensation'

973
In examining the mental state of a patient
A a dejected posture suggests depressive illness
B a girl's repetitive worry that she may be pregnant, although she knows quite well she has not had sexual intercourse, implies that she has a delusion
C rapid speech, punctuated by puns and rhymes, occurs in schizophrenia
D he is hallucinated if he describes furniture as taking on the shape of a menacing person
E testing recent memory is a useful way of assessing intellectual function

974
Psychoneurosis
A is more easily accepted as a diagnosis by patients in the lower social classes
B is the most common type of psychiatric disorder encountered in general practice
C does not necessarily demand treatment
D takes many forms, of which anxiety is the least common
E is usually preceded by intrapersonal subjective tension

975
In a case of anxiety neurosis
A hereditary factors play a major part in the genesis of the disease
B prolonged insecurity in childhood is more likely to be aetiologically relevant than an isolated trauma in early life
C periodical exacerbation may be expected at times of social setback
D hypochondriasis is often found
E there is a serious risk of suicide

976
In the treatment of anxiety neurosis
A with somatic symptoms it is best simply to tell the patient that there is nothing wrong with him
B diazepam may be needed to reduce distress before psychotherapy can be effective
C the doctor should maintain silence until the end of a psychotherapeutic interview
D behaviour therapy is often effective in a patient with a specific phobia e.g. of air journeys
E if a patient confronts and masters a painful situation, there is likely to be a temporary exacerbation of symptoms

977
Hysterical symptoms
A are more likely to occur in association with educational disadvantage
B may take a form determined by identification with another person
C include deafness
D must be distinguished from a fugue state, which indicates a psychotic illness
E are unlikely to appear for the first time in adult life in a previously stable person

978
Patients suffering from anorexia nervosa
A are usually reluctant to undertake any form of physical activity
B are nearly always profoundly depressed
C are afraid of growing up
D sometimes deliberately induce vomiting
E require in-patient treatment

979

Obsessive-compulsive symptoms

A are often found in several members of the same family

B may take the form of ruminations

C are recognised as absurd by the patient

D respond well to treatment

E only carry a serious risk of suicide if they have led to depression

980

A depressive psychoneurosis

A is usually unrelated to any personal setback

B is often unresponsive to out-patient treatment

C commonly develops after influenza

D is often admixed with anxiety reaction

E when accompanied by sleep disturbance and constipation, may require treatment with antidepressive drugs

981

In a phobic neurosis

A the patient's fear is firmly related to a precise stimulus

B the phobic object is to some extent alarming to most normal people

C there may be fear of open spaces

D the patient nearly always seeks advice about his phobia early in the illness

E improvement cannot be expected unless the patient can avoid all exposure to the phobic object or situation

982

The following statements about personality disorder are correct:

A The persistent abnormality of behaviour is necessarily antisocial

B Psychopaths are more socially destructive than hysterical people

C An obsessional person, though overcareful and meticulous, is quite ready to change his opinion on a subject without difficulty

D A schizoid person is rigid and brittle

E A hysterical disorder shows itself by selfishness and carelessness of the opinion of other people

983

A sociopath

A has a serious defect in the capacity for feeling

B is always aggressive

C indulges in monotonously repetitive antisocial behaviour

D is loyal to other sociopaths

E may be superficially likeable and charming

984

Alcohol addiction

A is difficult to treat successfully even if the patient is distressed by his abnormality

B carries an increased risk of suicide

C is a greater problem in Scotland than in England

D may be uncovered as a result of an unexpected hospital admission

E may be usefully treated by disulfiram

985

Addiction to

A morphine may cause a sensation of insects crawling under the skin

B cocaine occurs only if the drug is taken as snuff

C LSD can lead to suicide

D barbiturates can cause ataxia

E amphetamine may cause a syndrome indistinguishable from paranoid schizophrenia

986

Features of a depressive illness include

A inability to make decisions

B association with psychosomatic disease such as asthma

C an overscrupulous rigid personality

D a high incidence in the young

E a fear of impending insanity

987

A patient suffering from schizophrenia

A tends to believe that he is being punished for his wrong-doings

B feels that other people put thoughts into his mind

C when paranoid, may require compulsory admission to hospital by means of an emergency order

D may be highly intelligent

E has a definitely better prognosis if treated with a phenothiazine

988

In the elderly

A anxiety states are particularly difficult to alleviate

B any change of scene is poorly tolerated

C isolation from other people should be advised if they are disturbed

D chloral hydrate is of particular value if sleep is disturbed

E chlorpromazine is especially likely to produce postural dizziness

CHAPTER SIXTEEN

989

Self-poisoning

A is more common in dense conurbations than in rural communities

B has increased approximately three-fold in the past thirty years

C is a term which includes all forms of suicidal poisoning

D is most often with the benzodiazepine group of drugs

E often occurs in a setting of poverty and alcoholism

990

Essential measures in the immediate management of all cases of acute poisoning include

A precise identification of the poison

B administration of an antidote

C maintenance of a clear airway

D attempts to enhance the elimination of the poison

E prophylactic antibiotic therapy

991

Gastric lavage

A is unlikely to be useful if eight hours have elapsed since an overdose of salicylate was taken

B is contra-indicated if the patient has taken paraffin oil

C is safer than the induction of vomiting in a semi-conscious patient

D should be carried out with a solution of sodium bicarbonate in salicylate poisoning

E may yield worthwhile recovery of a tricyclic antidepressant up to 12 hours after ingestion

992

When a stomach tube is passed in a patient suffering from self-poisoning

A the patient should be lying on his left side

B the foot of the bed should be raised

C who is deeply unconscious, a cuffed endotracheal tube must be inserted

D tepid water should be introduced into the stomach before the gastric contents are aspirated

E its position in the stomach should always be verified by radiography

993
In a patient suffering from self-poisoning, hypothermia
A is not dangerous unless the rectal temperature is below 35°C
B may require treatment with hydrocortisone
C increases the oxygen demands of the tissues
D can cause hypotension
E should be treated by active reheating if the core temperature is below 32°C

994
Barbiturate poisoning should be categorised as severe if
A there is no response to maximal painful stimulation
B the blood barbiturate concentration is above 5mg/100 ml
C the pupils are dilated
D the minute volume of expired air is less than four litres
E the tendon reflexes are diminished

995
In poisoning with
A nitrazepam profound hypotension is a recognised finding
B methaqualone and diphenhydramine (Mandrax) papilloedema may be found
C glutethimide there is considerable variation in the conscious level
D barbiturates considerable tachycardia is to be expected
E morphine the pupils are widely dilated

996
Recognised findings in amitriptyline poisoning include
A cardiac arrhythmias
B convulsions
C fixed dilated pupils
D profuse salivation
E sluggish reflexes

997
In a patient who has taken a large overdose of salicylate
A the arterial blood pH first rises above, then falls below, normal
B hypokalaemia is a recognised finding
C severe dehydration can be expected to develop
D proteinuria is of no long term significance
E haematemesis from gastric erosions is the most common cause of death

998
The treatment of poisoning with
A salicylate should include assisted ventilation
B imipramine may need to include physostigmine
C paracetamol includes intravenous administration of atropine
D cyanide includes intravenous administration of cobalt edetate
E opiates includes intravenous administration of naloxone

999
Recognised manifestations of paracetamol poisoning include
A bronchospasm
B hypoglycaemia
C renal failure
D bradycardia
E liver failure

1000
Recognised manifestations of carbon monoxide poisoning include
A extensor plantar responses
B hypotension
C cardiac arrhythmias
D cyanosis
E cutaneous bullae

1001
Children
A could be largely protected from accidental poisoning if tablets were not sugar coated
B are less likely than adults to develop dangerous cardiac arrhythmias if poisoned with a tricyclic antidepressant drug
C are more susceptible than adults to the severe acid-base disturbances of salicylate poisoning
D are at special risk if poisoned with iron salts
E who swallow detergents rarely survive

1002
Psychiatric assessment in cases of self-poisoning
A is not necessary unless there is obvious major psychiatric disturbance
B should be carried out as soon as possible after the act
C may be misleading if the patient discusses the episode with his relatives beforehand
D has not been shown to influence the incidence of subsequent acts of self-poisoning
E is not necessary if the self-poisoning seems to have been accidental

CHAPTER SEVENTEEN

1003
The following statements about diseases in the tropics are correct:
A Food taboos contribute to the incidence of malnutrition
B Amoebiasis is the most important cause of the high infant mortality in the tropics
C Yellow fever has been controlled by vaccination
D Poliomyelitis in an endemic area mostly affects middle aged adults
E The eradication of smallpox in man is made more difficult by the fact that monkeys are susceptible to the disease

1004
The following statements about geographical influences on disease are correct:
A The causes of heart disease in the tropics do not differ significantly from those in temperate climates
B Primary arteritis of the aorta and its main branches is relatively common in S.E. Asia
C Phlebitis of uncertain origin occurs especially in tropical Africa
D Worms are a recognised cause of respiratory diseases in S.E. Asia
E Appendicitis is commoner in the tropics because of the added hazard of whipworm infection

1005
The following diseases are commoner in many rural parts of the tropics than in temperate zones:
A chronic bronchitis
B varicose veins
C asthma
D coronary heart disease
E pericarditis

1006
Tropical sprue
A is due primarily to sensitivity to rice protein
B is associated with gross overpopulation of the jejunum by *Staphylococcus aureus*
C may lead to hypomagnesaemia
D should be treated with a high lactose diet
E should be treated with oral tetracycline

1007
Recognised clinical features of tropical sprue include
A tetany
B cheilosis
C generalised pigmentation
D a scaphoid abdomen
E nocturia

1008
Recognised causes of chronic anaemia among Negroes in the tropics include
A amoebiasis
B homozygous α-thalassaemia
C haemoglobin SS disease
D malaria
E ascariasis

1009
G6PD deficiency
A is inherited as an X-linked recessive disorder
B does not affect females
C causes haemolysis which may be self limiting because only red cells over a certain age are affected
D takes a more serious form in Caucasians than in Negroes
E can be detected by electrophoretic analysis of haemoglobin

1010
In sickle cell disease and trait
A the presence of the haemoglobin genotype SC causes less disability than SS
B the presence of the haemoglobin genotype AS can be diagnosed by microscopic examination of a stained blood film
C a characteristic symptom of the disease in the first two years of life is pain in the fingers and toes
D the associated bossing of the head is due to malabsorption of vitamin D
E aseptic necrosis of the femoral head is a recognised complication in adults

1011
The following statements about haemoglobin and its variants are correct:
A Haemoglobin SS is typically associated with anaemia from birth
B The persistence of haemoglobin F in adults carrying the haemoglobin S gene worsens the prognosis
C Reoxygenation can depolymerise tactoids
D The alpha chains are identical in haemoglobins A, A_2 and F
E The possession of haemoglobin $α2ß2$ is typically associated with haemolytic anaemia

1012
Recognised clinical features of sickle cell disease include
A fever
B nephrolithiasis
C ulceration of the mouth
D fat embolism
E mesenteric infarction

1013
Features which are common to beta thalassaemia major and minor include
A a Mongoloid facies
B massive hepato-splenomegaly
C hypochromic anaemia
D a positive family history
E a progression to haemosiderosis

1014
Beta thalassaemia major
A is characterised by an abnormal aminoacid structure of the polypeptide chain
of haemoglobin
B when recognised allows the confident
prediction of raised levels of
haemoglobin F in both parents
C causes inability to synthesise
haemoglobin A
D should be treated by long-term oral iron
therapy
E constitutes an absolute contra-
indication to splenectomy

1015
In Burkitt's lymphoma
A the typical presentation is a generalised
lymphadenopathy
B loosening of the teeth is an early
feature of mandibular involvement
C a tumour of the maxilla may present
as exophthalmos
D climatic conditions are thought to affect
the development of the disease
E radiotherapy is the treatment of choice

1016
Tropical pyomyositis
A usually follows tropical phlebitis
B predominantly affects muscles of the
pectoral girdle and upper arms
C occurs mostly in India
D causes abscesses which should be
incised
E is associated with blood eosinophilia

1017
During acclimatisation to heat
A maximal adjustment takes 10-14 days
B very little exercise should be taken
C the blood volume falls because of
increased sweating
D aldosterone secretion increases
E the salt content of sweat falls

1018
Prickly heat
A causes a fine, papular urticarial rash
B is due to photo-sensitisation
C should be treated with a long-acting
antihistamine
D is improved by moving the patient to a
cool environment
E is improved by encouraging gustatory
sweating (e.g. by eating curry)

1019
Recognised clinical features of heat
exhaustion include
A thirst
B muscular cramps
C marked polyuria
D a flushed sweaty skin
E tachycardia

1020
Heat hyperpyrexia
A is a recognised sequel of extensive
prickly heat
B occurs only in subjects who have been
exposed to direct sunshine
C may occur without warning
D is always associated with absence of
sweating
E should be treated by reducing the
temperature slowly

1021
The following statements are correct:
A Multifocal malignant melanomata of
the skin result from prolonged exposure
to sunshine
B Mountain sickness is almost unknown
at altitudes below 15000 feet (4575 m)
C Acute pulmonary oedema may result
from rapid ascent to high altitudes
D Papilloedema may result from ascent to
high altitudes
E An ambient temperature of –5°C is
more likely to cause frostbite at high
altitudes than at sea level

1022
The *Plasmodia* which cause malaria in
man
A are transmitted solely through the bite
of anopheline mosquitoes
B consist of four major species
C undergo a sexual cycle in the 6–12
days between infection and the onset
of the first symptoms
D cause the first symptoms through the
liberation of sporozoites from ruptured
oocysts
E all have a persistent exo-erythrocytic
phase except *P. falciparum*

1023
The following statements about the life cycle of the malarial parasite are correct:
A Sporozoites inoculated by the mosquito disappear from the blood within half-an-hour
B All plasmodia first multiply in the liver except *P. falciparum*
C Merozoites re-entering red cells may undergo sexual or asexual development
D The erythrocytic (asexual) cycle occurs in all species except *P. falciparum*
E Fertilisation of the female gamete occurs in the stomach of the mosquito

1024
Recognised features of *P. falciparum* malaria include
A symptoms due to blocking of capillaries by infected red cells
B a higher level of fever than in the other three types
C coma
D resistance to chloroquine in certain regions
E rapid intravascular haemolysis

1025
Drugs which are effective in the initial stages of treatment of an overt attack of vivax malaria include
A quinine
B proguanil
C amodiaquine
D chloroquine
E pyrimethamine

1026
The tropical splenomegaly syndrome
A is characterised by gross splenomegaly
B occurs in areas of malarial hyperendemicity
C may be confused with myelomatosis as a result of plasmacytosis in blood and bone marrow
D can be diagnosed by finding IgM aggregates in the Kupffer cells in a liver biopsy
E is best treated by splenectomy

1027
Amoebic dysentery
A is endemic in all continents
B has an incubation period of 7–10 days
C characteristically presents with acute diarrhoea
D shows a typical sigmoidoscopic appearance
E affects the rectum more extensively than other parts of the alimentary tract

1028
Recognised complications of amoebiasis include
A severe intestinal haemorrhage
B expectoration of the contents of a liver abscess
C radiographic filling defect in the colon resembling carcinoma
D brain abscess
E ulceration of the wound following appendicectomy

1029
In the diagnosis and treatment of amoebiasis
A vegetative amoebae are unlikely to be found in the stools if mucus is present
B active *E. histolytica* are identified by ingested red cells and the protrusion of pseudopodia containing clear ectoplasm
C a hepatic abscess may be located by ultrasonic scanning
D the contents of an amoebic liver abscess are characterised by the presence of cysts
E hepatic involvement may be effectively treated by metronidazole 800 mg t.i.d. for 2 days

1030
In giardiasis
A the infection is in the duodenum and jejunum
B the larvae enter through the skin of the feet
C malabsorption is a recognised feature
D the organism may be obtained by jejunal aspiration
E thiabendazole is the treatment of choice

1031
In kala azar
A transmission is by mosquitoes
B the incubation period may be several years
C massive hepatomegaly and slight splenomegaly are characteristic
D groups of characteristic ovoid bodies occur in the reticulo-endothelial cells of the bone marrow
E metronidazole is the drug of choice in treatment

1032
The following statements about visceral leishmaniasis are correct:
A It is exclusively a disease of man
B Lymphadenopathy may be the only abnormal sign
C Leucocytosis fluctuates in parallel with the fever
D The serum concentration of IgG is typically raised
E Cirrhosis of the liver is a common complication

1033
Leishmaniasis of the skin
A due to *L. donovani* may affect any part of the skin
B causes an indurated ulcer up to 10cm diameter
C is accompanied by severe toxaemia
D can be prevented by inoculation with living *L. tropica*
E is accompanied by a positive leishmanin skin test if the lesions are sufficiently widespread

1034
Cutaneous leishmaniasis due to *L. tropica*
A is part of a widespread zoonosis
B involves only those areas of skin which are covered by clothing
C produces papules which are surrounded by tiny satellite lesions
D may cause ulceration of the nose and upper lip
E cannot be identified by artificial culture of the causative organism

1035
In S. American leishmaniasis
A *L. Braziliensis* may cause ulceration of the nasal or oral mucosa
B *L. Mexicana* causes painful ulcers in the groins of workers gathering chicle
C *L. Peruviana* causes massive splenomegaly and leucopenia
D all three of the above species are spread from animals by insects
E sodium stibogluconate by injection is the treatment of choice

1036
African trypanosomiasis
A can be prevented in West Africa for up to 6 months by a single intramuscular injection of 250 mg pentamidine
B is indirectly a cause of protein malnutrition
C is spread to man by cattle ticks
D causes a skin lesion resembling a chancre
E is most easily diagnosed by blood culture

1037
Recognised features of infection by Trypanosoma (Trypanozoon) brucei *(T. (T.) b.) gambiense* include.
A a reservoir in animals including cattle
B inversion of sleep rhythm as an early symptom
C lymphadenopathy
D the presence of trypanosomes in a lymph node aspirate
E an improvement of the neurological features in response to treatment with an antimony compound

1038
In American trypanosomiasis (Chagas' disease)
A dogs and cats are the most important animal hosts
B infection is transmitted to man through the bites, scratches and licks of domestic pets
C a punched out, indolent ulcer marks the site of entry
D there is a persistent dry cough in the febrile invasion stage
E cardiomyopathy may result in sudden death

1039
Infection by *Toxoplasma gondii*
A is acquired by inhalation of dust
   containing ova
B in its congenital form causes
   developmental cardiac defects
C in its acquired form may present with
   generalised lymphadenopathy
D is a recognised cause of chorioretinitis
E can be confirmed by serological tests

1040
Granuloma venereum
A is clinically manifest only in the male
B spreads widely as serpiginous ulcers in
   moist areas around the scrotum
C causes local tender lymphadenopathy
D is confirmed by the demonstration of
   Donovan bodies in mononuclear cells
   of the lesion
E responds to treatment with
   metronidazole

1041
Bartonellosis
A is widespread throughout the coastal
   areas of South America
B has a gradual onset with a peak of
   fever about the tenth day
C typically causes severe haemolysis
D can be confirmed by finding Bartonellae
   in red cells in a stained blood smear
E may be followed in a month or more by
   characteristic cherry-red cutaneous
   nodules on the head and limbs

1042
Melioidosis
A is a systemic fungal infection derived
   from mouldy hay
B causes fever and pneumonia
C produces only minimal changes in the
   chest radiograph
D may be diagnosed by culture of pus
   from a subcutaneous abscess
E is unresponsive to antibiotics

1043
Recognised features of leprosy include
A dermal lesions with a cellular response
   directly proportional to the number of
   organisms present
B spread through close association with a
   patient with the tuberculoid form
C failure of the organism to grow on
   artificial media
D an incubation period of 2-5 years
E spontaneous healing of the earliest
   macular lesion

1044
**The macular lesions of lepromatous
leprosy are characterised by**
A their small size
B a symmetrical distribution
C a predilection for the extensor surface
   of the arms and fronts of the legs
D slightly raised, clearcut margins
E impairment of appreciation of light
   touch over the lesions

1045
**Characteristic features of tuberculoid
leprosy include**
A a predilection for the face and ears
B palpable thickening of nerves
C a high risk of developing erythema
   nodosum leprosum
D a positive smear from the depths of a
   skin slit
E a positive lepromin test

1046
A type 2 lepra reaction
A is due to the deposition of immune
   complexes
B occurs most often in patients with
   active cell-mediated immunity
C can be treated effectively with
   thalidomide
D can include iritis
E is most often precipitated by erratic
   treatment with dapsone

1047
The following statements about leprosy are correct:
A The organism can be found in nasal mucus in the lepromatous form
B The nodular lesions of the lepromatous form are swellings on infected peripheral nerves
C Gynaecomastia is a recognised complication
D The mucous membranes of the upper respiratory tract may ulcerate
E The combination of 5th and 7th cranial nerve damage may lead to blindness

1048
In the treatment of leprosy
A there is a danger of resistance to dapsone arising in some lepromatous cases
B rifampicin produces quicker clinical improvement than dapsone
C a specific vaccine is now available
D clofazimine darkens the colour of the patient's skin
E the disease tends to disappear with improvement in socio-economic conditions

1049
In infections due to *Vibrio cholerae*
A the incubation period may be only a few hours
B the majority of patients suffer severe symptoms
C after evacuating the faecal contents of the gut, the stools consist of clear fluid containing mucus
D the diarrhoea is associated with severe periumbilical colic
E death may result from loss of fluid into the dilated bowel without diarrhoea

1050
In the treatment of cholera
A a rapid blood transfusion should be given if the blood pressure falls
B vomiting precludes the use of nasogastric rehydration
C a severe case should receive intravenous fluids run in as fast as possible
D glucose added to oral fluids promotes electrolyte absorption
E tetracycline given for 3 days reduces the duration of excretion of vibrios

1051
The following statements about anthrax are correct:
A The spores remain viable in soil for years
B It is a recognised occupational disease of gardeners
C A malignant pustule on the face is very painful
D Eating infected meat may cause fatal gastroenteritis
E Penicillin therapy is effective

1052
Plague due to *Yersinia pestis*
A spread among the Philistines in Old Testament times (*I Samuel,* Chapters 5 and 6)
B is spread to man through the sole agency of the rat flea
C causes painful buboes draining the area of the primary skin infection
D is best treated with streptomycin
E is best confirmed in a suspicious case by examining a methylene blue-stained smear of aspirate from a bubo

1053
Recognised features of tularaemia include
A gradual onset of fever
B an inflammatory swelling at the portal of entry
C enlargement of regional lymph nodes
D leucopenia
E positive blood culture for *Yersinia tularensis*

1054
In a case of chancroid
A there is gross enlargement of the labia (esthiomene)
B there are multiple penile lesions varying from a small red papule to a painful ulcer
C systemic symptoms are absent
D it is important to make dark ground examinations of pus from the lesion
E the diagnosis may be established by examining a lymph node aspirate

1055
Infection by *Treponema pertenue* results in
A serological changes similar to those of syphilis
B a prostrating illness in the primary stage
C visceral lesions resembling gummata
D a primary lesion usually on the face
E hypertrophic periosteal lesions

1056
Yaws
A is spread from case to case by a reduviid bug
B has an incubation period of 2–5 days
C results in a punched-out 'tissue paper' scar at the site of the healed 'mother yaw'
D gives rise to a secondary eruption consisting of papillomata covered with a whitish-yellow exudate
E can be cured in most active cases by two intramuscular injections of 750 mg of procaine benzylpenicillin at an interval of one week

1057
Endemic (non-venereal) syphilis
A is caused by *Treponema carateum*
B prevails in families whose social conditions are poor
C sometimes spreads by the use of common drinking vessels
D typically leads to congenital disease in the infants of infected mothers
E causes widespread neurological disease in affected communities

1058
Pinta
A is endemic in tropical Africa
B is due to fungal infection
C causes a generalised eruption of pinkish, slightly scaly macules and miliary papules 5–12 months after the primary lesion
D leads eventually to atrophic and depigmented skin patches
E is best treated with griseofulvin

1059
Louse-borne relapsing fever
A is transmitted through skin from infected lice crushed by scratching
B is characterised by febrile periods of sudden onset and ending by crisis
C is confirmed by the demonstration of *Spirillum minus* in exudate from the eschar
D may be treated successfully with a single oral dose of doxycycline
E treated successfully by chemotherapy is inevitably complicated by a Jarisch-Herxheimer reaction

1060
In tick-borne relapsing fever
A the infection can be transmitted congenitally in ticks
B man is the only known mammalian host
C optic atrophy is a recognised complication
D the causative agent (*Borrelia duttoni*) may be demonstrable in a stained blood film
E the treatment of choice is procaine penicillin by intramuscular injection

1061
Of the two varieties of rat-bite fever, that due to *Streptobacillus moniliformis* is distinguished by
A a liability also to be spread by the rat flea
B an inflammatory reaction at the site of the bite which develops from 5–21 days after initial healing
C recurrent bouts of fever lasting 24–48 hours for several weeks
D painful arthritis
E a false positive serological test for syphilis

1062
Tropical ulcer
A follows minor injury in those living in a poor state of hygiene, health and nutrition
B is associated with infection by diphtheroid organisms
C occurs most commonly on the face
D starts as a bleb filled with sanguineous fluid
E may become carcinomatous

1063
Infections due to arboviruses
A occur predominantly in the tropics
B are the cause of over 80 different diseases in man
C are divided into Groups A, B and C on the basis of neurotropic, viscerotropic or other activity
D are transmitted to man from trees and shrubs by infected pollen
E are the cause of liver damage in Kyasanur Forest Disease

1064
The following statements about yellow fever are correct:
A South East Asia is one of the main endemic areas
B Urban infection is transmitted from man to man by *Aedes aegypti*
C Rural infection may be derived from monkeys via *Aedes simpsoni*
D An infected mosquito dies within three weeks of ingesting the virus
E Many inhabitants of endemic areas acquire immunity from subclinical infections

1065
In yellow fever
A the incubation period is 3–6 weeks
B jaundice precedes fever
C proteinuria may occur even in the absence of jaundice
D a polymorphonuclear leucocytosis distinguishes the disease from other types of viral hepatitis
E an effective vaccine is not yet available

1066
In sandfly fever
A the disease is transmitted to man from its natural host the desert rat
B the sandfly remains infective for life
C some cross immunity develops with other members of the B group of arboviruses, including yellow fever
D fever of shorter duration and the absence of a rash distinguish the illness from dengue
E an ordinary mosquito net sprayed with insecticide is an ineffective prophylactic because the sandfly is so tiny

1067
Japanese B encephalitis
A is at present confined to the Japanese mainland
B is acquired by eating undercooked or raw fresh water crustacea
C leaves no permanent neurological sequelae
D may be manifest as meningitis only without clinical evidence of encephalitis
E is most common, in endemic areas, as a subclinical infection

1068
Rabies
A is maintained in Europe from a reservoir of infection in foxes
B typically affects man as a result of a lick or a bite from a dog
C cannot be transmitted by cats
D has an incubation period ranging from nine days to many months
E is almost invariably fatal

1069
The following statements about rabies are correct:
A A bite by a rabid animal will cause rabies unless effective prophylactic action is taken
B Bites on the head and neck have the shortest incubation period
C Violent spasms of the inspiratory muscles provoked by attempts to drink are characteristic of the disease
D Human antirabies immunoglobulin is unobtainable because affected patients do not survive
E Duck egg vaccine carries a greater risk of neuroparalysis than Semple-type vaccine

1070
In Lassa fever
A recognised outbreaks have been limited to S. America
B there is a reservoir of infection in dogs
C case to case transmission has occurred
D adherent yellow exudates on the pharynx are particularly characteristic
E evidence of subclinical infection has not yet been found

1071
In Marburg disease
A the onset of fever is sudden
B the rash is maculo-papular in type
C the lymph nodes may be enlarged
D haemorrhagic phenomena, when they occur, are due to hepatic damage causing failure of prothrombin production
E a fatal encephalitis may develop

1072
Lymphogranuloma inguinale
A is due to infection by *Wuchereria bancrofti*
B heals quickly with little scar formation after early treatment with penicillin
C leads to the discharge of thick, glairy fluid from affected lymph nodes
D can be confirmed by a positive skin reaction to the Dmelcos vaccine
E may cause rectal stricture

1073
In trachoma
A infection may occur at birth
B follicular conjunctivitis of the upper lid is an early ophthalmic feature
C blindness is usually the result of cataract
D treatment with oral sulphonamide combined with tetracycline eye drops may give good results
E the infective organism can be demonstrated in a conjunctival snip

1074
The insect vectors which transmit rickettsiae causing different types of typhus fever include
A fleas
B sandflies
C mites
D bed bugs
E mosquitoes

1075
The mammalian reservoir from which infection by Rickettsiae is derived is
A man in endemic typhus
B the rat in epidemic typhus
C rodents and dogs in Rocky Mountain spotted fever
D cattle in African tick-borne typhus
E mice in rickettsialpox

1076
The following statements about the various forms of typhus fever are correct:
A Rickettsiae characteristically parasitise the endothelium of small blood vessels
B In epidemic typhus an eschar with regional lymphadenopathy characteristically forms at the portal of entry
C In scrub typhus the brain is particularly prone to attack
D In tick typhus, unlike other forms, the rash starts peripherally
E Tetracycline is effective in the treatment of all rickettsial infections

1077
Q fever is
A due to infection by *Coxiella burneti*
B known to affect farm animals
C typically spread to man by tick bites
D a recognised cause of infective endocarditis
E characterised by the development of agglutinins to both *Proteus OX 19* and *OXK* (positive Weil-Felix reaction)

1078
The following statements are correct about all types of schistosomiasis:
A Cercariae are passed in the urine and/or stool
B The parasite multiplies in a freshwater snail
C Itchy papules and vesicles occur at the site of primary infection
D A single dose of hycanthone is effective treatment
E The introduction of the water snake *Enhydrina schistosa* into infected lakes and rivers destroys the intermediary snail host

1079
Infection with *Schistosoma haematobium*
A is widespread in Africa and the Middle East
B is confined to the urinary tract
C causes the appearance of 'sandy patches' visible on cystoscopy
D characteristically causes painless terminal haematuria as an early symptom
E disappears spontaneously within six months after the patient has left the endemic region

1080
Infection with *Schistosoma mansoni*
A predominantly involves the ileum
B occurs in a wide range of mammalian hosts besides man
C may cause the formation of large pedunculated papillomata in the bowel
D after ten years or so leads to an increasingly serious risk of malignant change in the bowel
E may lead to cor pulmonale

1081
Infection with *Schistosoma japonicum*
A is not confined to Japan
B occurs as a result of eating raw or inadequately cooked freshwater crustacea
C can cause Jacksonian epilepsy
D may give rise to severe abdominal pain and diarrhoea
E is best confirmed by intradermal skin testing

1082
All the flukes which infect the bile duct in man
A are endemic in the Far East only
B have snails as an intermediate host
C have freshwater fish as a second intermediate host
D can cause cholangitis
E produce ova which can be found in duodenal aspirate

1083
Fasciolopsiasis
A is a disease of sheep
B infects man through ingestion of uncooked water plants
C presents clinically with obstructive jaundice
D is diagnosed by detecting metacercariae in the stools
E can be treated effectively with piperazine

1084
Infection with *Taenia solium*
A can only occur in man as a result of eating undercooked beef
B is usually identified by finding the characteristic ova in the stools
C may progress to cysticercosis if ova enter the stomach
D is nearly always associated with extensive intracranial calcification in patients developing epilepsy
E is best treated with niclosamide

1085
In hydatid disease
A man is infected by ova from sheep faeces carried by a dog
B embryos liberated from ingested ova enter the portal blood stream
C the cyst expands rapidly
D surgical drainage of the cyst is preferable to removal
E the right lobe of the liver is involved in about 75 per cent of cases

1086
Infection with threadworms
A is common in children
B is best detected by searching for ova in the stools
C is more likely to be eradicated if the whole family is treated simultaneously
D causes severe abdominal pain
E may respond to treatment with piperazine

1087
Toxocara canis infection
A is acquired through the skin
B is found in adults more commonly than
   in children
C may cause asthma in man
D may cause a granuloma in the eye
   which resembles a neoplasm
E is best treated with tetrachloroethylene

1088
Ascaris lumbricoides
A ova are not infective until their
   contained embryos have developed
B causes pneumonia and eosinophilia if
   infection is heavy
C may be vomited by an infected patient
D is a recognised cause of bile-duct
   obstruction
E infection is effectively treated with filix
   mas

1089
The following clinical manifestations
should arouse a suspicion of infection
with Ancylostoma duodenale in an
endemic area:
A patchy pulmonary consolidation with
   eosinophilia
B vomiting with epigastric pain
C obstructive jaundice
D larva migrans
E severe anaemia

1090
Strongyloidiasis
A may cause itching during invasion of
   the skin
B may cause linear urticaria around the
   anus
C produces no abdominal symptoms
D is best diagnosed by finding ova of *S.*
   stercoralis in the fresh stool
E is best treated with thiabendazole

1091
Infection with Trichinella spiralis
A is acquired from contact with rats'
   urine
B is a febrile illness
C causes oedema of the face
D is one of the few helminth infections
   which does not produce eosinophilia
E is confirmed diagnostically by finding
   the characteristic ova in the stools

1092
Involvement of the eye is a recognised
feature of helminthic infections by
A *Loa loa*
B *Gnathostoma spinigerum*
C *Necator americanus*
D *Onchocerca volvulus*
E *Schistosoma japonicum*

1093
The organism can be identified in a wet
blood film taken from a patient infected
with
A *Trichinella spiralis*
B *Onchocerca volvulus*
C *Loa loa*
D *Dipetalonema perstans*
E *Brugia malayi*

1094
Infection with Wuchereria bancrofti
A is characterised by the entry of
   microfilariae into the blood stream by
   night in the case of the strain
   transmitted by *Culex fatigans*
B causes fever with tenderness along
   inflamed lymphatic vessels
C leads to elephantiasis within one or
   two years
D may cause chylous ascites
E is best treated with levamisole

1095
Onchocerciasis
A is transmitted by the bite of the tsetse
   fly
B can be prevented by drainage of ponds
   and areas of stagnant water around
   dwellings
C causes transient Calabar swellings
   before the onchocercoma develops
D is a recognised cause of orchitis
E is best diagnosed by a complement
   fixation test if no nodule is available for
   biopsy

F

1096

Loiasis is

A transmitted by the day biting fly Chrysops

B endemic in and around equatorial rain forests

C typically accompanied by eosinophilia

D cured by treatment with diethylcarbamazine

E sometimes complicated by fever, malaise and joint and muscle pains during curative chemotherapy

1097

In dracontiasis

A infection is transmitted by drinking water containing ova discharged by the adult worm

B the female worm takes at least 9 months to grow over a metre in length before emerging

C redness, tenderness and vesicle formation precede emergence of the head through the skin of the lower leg

D systemic symptoms are absent unless secondary infection occurs

E the female worm may calcify and be visible in a radiograph

1098

The following statements about histoplasmosis are correct:

A The survival of spores outside the body is of brief duration

B Pulmonary infections characteristically run a malignant course

C Addison's disease is a recognised sequel to adrenal involvement

D *Histoplasma duboisii* occurs in tropical Africa

E Treatment with tetracycline is curative

1099

The following statements about mycetoma are correct:

A The disease is caused by several varieties of both *Maduromycetoma* and aerobic *Actinomycetecea*

B The disease consists of a chronic fibrosing granuloma

C An exquisitely painful ulcer appears at the site of inoculation by a thorn

D Amputation, hitherto necessary, has been obviated by treatment with cotrimoxazole

E Bone damage is common

1100

In a patient who has been bitten by an adder (*Vipera berus*)

A a cruciate incision should be made at the site of the bite

B the affected part should be immobilised as for a fracture

C a venous tourniquet should be applied and released briefly every 30 minutes

D paroxysms of hypertension are a recognised complication

E specific Zagreb antivenom should be given in all cases

PART TWO

Section 1
In Part Two (Questions 1101–1200) the questions are based on either Macleod's *Clinical Examination* (prefixed by the letter M) or Davidson's *Principles and Practice of Medicine*. In Section 1 the questions are of the Independent True/False type as in Part One.

Section I

M 1101
Orthopnoea is a recognised manifestation of
A spontaneous pneumothorax
B intrapleural haemorrhage
C massive pulmonary embolism
D left ventricular failure
E emphysema

M 1102
The following features may be of diagnostic significance in a patient complaining of dyspnoea:
A the severity of the dyspnoea
B a bruit over the thyroid gland
C a history of tetany
D ptosis of variable severity
E displacement of the apex beat

M 1103
In a patient with obstructive jaundice
A the colour of the urine resembles that of beer
B the colour of the skin depends on the depth and duration of jaundice
C scratch marks due to pruritus indicate that the obstruction is extra-hepatic
D bilirubin is excreted in the urine attached to albumin
E a yellow froth is easily produced when the urine is shaken

M 1104
Anthropometric examination will show that
A sitting height is greater than pubis to ground height in hypogonadism
B sitting height is less than pubis to ground height in Marfan's syndrome
C the arm span is greater than twice the sitting height in achondroplasia
D there is usually some reduction of pubis to ground height in rickets
E the sitting height of a normal young adult may be less at the end of the day than in the morning

M 1105
In the nails
A transverse grooves are suggestive of hypoalbuminaemia
B small white isolated patches are a sign of liver disease
C splinter haemorrhages are seen occasionally in normal subjects
D an increase in the normal convexity may be due to iron deficiency
E severe pitting and deformity associated with swelling of the terminal interphalangeal joints are suggestive of psoriasis

M 1106
The teeth
A normally number 36 in adults
B may be discoloured yellow in children with severe neonatal jaundice
C have normally all erupted, except the third molars, by the age of 12 years
D become grey in fluorosis
E are hypoplastic in juvenile hypoparathyroidism

M 1107
In the examination of lymph nodes
A supraclavicular nodes should be felt from behind
B the left hand is best used for exploring the left axilla
C para-aortic nodes cannot be felt by abdominal palpation
D it is often difficult to tell whether palpable inguinal nodes are pathological
E biopsy may help in the diagnosis of trypanosomiasis

M 1108
Symptoms which may give a clue to the cause of nasal obstruction include
A frontal headache
B toothache
C chronic mouth breathing
D haemoptysis
E alternating obstruction of the nasal airways'

M 1109
The following statements are correct:
A Sigmoidoscopy should precede barium enema examination in the investigation of large bowel disease
B In a patient with dysphagia, a normal barium swallow obviates the need for oesophagoscopy
C In acute abdominal conditions, plain X-rays of the abdomen should be obtained both in the erect and the lying positions
D Medicinal iron taken orally gives a false positive reaction when stools are tested for occult blood with the Hemoccult slide test
E Folic acid and vitamin B$_{12}$ absorption tests will not differentiate between disease of the jejunum and of the ileum

M 1110
The following findings are more likely to be of serious pathological significance in a one year old baby than in an adult:
A loss of weight
B a palpable left kidney
C extensor plantar response
D deviation of the trachea from the mid-line
E a palpable spleen

M 1111
A venous hum
A has been likened to the sound of a spinning top
B is abolished by pressure over the carotid sheath
C is an important clue to the presence of a persistent ductus arteriosus
D is exaggerated in the head-down position
E is characteristically accentuated in late systole

M 1112
In the examination of a child's heart, the following signs can be accepted as of no significance:
A sinus arrhythmia
B a soft diastolic murmur at the apex
C a venous hum
D a third heart sound at the apex
E a split second sound at the pulmonary area

1113
The primary chancre of syphilis
A can appear as early as two weeks after infection
B is typically painful
C usually ulcerates
D is associated with enlarged tender lymph nodes which often suppurate
E tends to heal spontaneously

1114
Vitamin K is required for the formation in the liver of
A Factor II
B Christmas factor
C Antihaemophilic factor
D Factor VII
E Factor X

1115
The following statements about vitamins of the B complex are correct:
A Pyridoxine may cure peripheral neuropathy arising during treatment with isoniazid
B Riboflavin deficiency is an important cause of death in malnourished rice-eaters in South East Asia
C Hydroxocobalamin by injection is of benefit in tropical ataxic neuropathy
D Megaloblastic anaemia in Crohn's disease of the terminal ileum is typically due to folate deficiency
E Vitamin B$_{12}$ deficiency can cause irreversible damage to peripheral nerves

1116
There is evidence that the ingestion of
A seeds of *Lathyrus sativus* causes the burning feet syndrome
B aflatoxin causes spastic paraplegia
C excessive amounts of vitamin A causes amblyopia
D cassava causes ataxia
E excessive amounts of vitamin E causes oxalate stones to form in the urinary tract

1117
The following statements are correct:
A Respiratory acidosis arises when the effective alveolar ventilation does not keep pace with the rate of production of CO_2
B The kidney responds to an increase in $PaCO_2$ by increasing bicarbonate excretion
C Over-ventilation during the course of assisted ventilation is a recognised cause of respiratory alkalosis
D Respiratory alkalosis is best treated by intravenous infusion of ammonium chloride
E During the assisted ventilation of a patient with hypercapnia through an endotracheal tube the concentration of oxygen used should not exceed 30 per cent

1118
In a patient with acute pulmonary oedema, morphine
A is contra-indicated if the heart failure is due to hypertension
B is best given intravenously
C should be given only if aminophylline produces no improvement
D may cause vomiting
E causes systemic venodilatation

1119
The electrocardiographic abnormalities found in patients with acute inferior myocardial infarction include
A ST segment elevation in lead aVF
B tall R waves in lead V1
C prominent Q waves in lead V6
D inverted T waves in lead II
E ST segment depression in leads V2-4

1120
Recognised fundal changes due to hypertension include
A micro-aneurysms
B flame-shaped haemorrhages
C arteriolar dilatation
D papilloedema
E soft exudates

1121
The following findings may be of value in determining the cause of a chronic cardiomyopathy:
A positive antinuclear factor test
B positive Paul-Bunnell test
C megacolon in a barium enema
D sinus tachycardia
E high serum iron concentration

1122
Chest pain
A is unusual in diaphragmatic pleurisy
B due to tracheitis is made worse by deep breathing
C exacerbated by deep breathing is pathognomonic of pleurisy
D due to pleurisy is caused by stretching of the visceral pleura
E may cause the cough to be short and suppressed in lobar pneumonia

1123
Recognised features of extrinsic allergic alveolitis include
A cellular exudate in the walls of alveoli and bronchioles
B decreased pulmonary compliance
C widespread rhonchi on auscultation
D an onset within a few minutes of exposure to the causative agent
E fever

1124
Bronchiectasis is
A a recognised sequel to bronchial obstruction
B a recognised complication of cystic fibrosis
C most often due to recurrent attacks of acute bronchitis
D found most frequently in the middle lobe
E typically associated with a morning cough productive of foetid sputum

1125
Bronchial adenomas
A occur in an older age group than do carcinomas
B are best treated by removal via a bronchoscope
C do not metastasise
D may present with diarrhoea
E characteristically present with recurrent haemoptysis

1126
Hiatus hernia
A of the paraoesophageal ('rolling') type is commoner than the oesophagogastric ('sliding') variety
B of the paraoesophageal variety is never associated with an incompetent· lower oesophageal sphincter
C occurs most often in elderly men
D of the oesophagogastric ('sliding') type is a recognised cause of oesophageal stricture
E is a recognised cause of iron deficiency anaemia

1127
Recognised unwanted effects of anticholinergic drugs include
A increased salivation
B diarrhoea
C retention of urine
D raised intraocular pressure
E blurring of vision

1128
In pancreatic insufficiency there is typically malabsorption of
A iron
B folate
C Vitamin D
D Vitamin B_{12}
E Vitamin A

1129
In normal man
A liver glycogen stores become exhausted within 24 hours of fasting
B the liver can convert lactate to glycogen
C approximately fifty per cent of endogenous glucose production is derived from the liver
D insulin suppresses lipolysis
E cortisol inhibits gluconeogenesis

1130
In the normal liver
A vitamin B_{12} is stored
B vitamin D_3 (cholecalciferol) is 25-hydroxylated
C paracetamol is inactivated
D microsomal enzyme activity is depressed by barbiturates
E about 50 per cent of ingested ethanol is metabolised

1131
The following diseases are correctly linked with a characteristic finding:
A Primary biliary cirrhosis and antimitochondrial antibody
B Hepatoma and alpha-fetoprotein
C Wilson's disease and increased serum caeruloplasmin concentration
D Liver disease in infancy and alpha$_1$-antitrypsin deficiency
E Haemochromatosis and low serum ferritin concentration

1132
Haemochromatosis
A is inherited as an autosomal recessive trait
B occurs twice as commonly in men as in women
C if untreated, typically leads to macronodular cirrhosis
D is usually associated with a normal serum ferritin concentration
E is best treated by injections of desferrioxamine

1133
Recognised associations of secondary haemosiderosis of the liver include
A sideroblastic anaemia
B chronic alcoholism
C multiple blood transfusions
D chronic pancreatitis
E excessive consumption of cheap wines

1134
Recognised causes of the nephrotic syndrome include
A diabetic nephropathy
B amyloid disease
C gold therapy
D proliferative glomerulonephritis
E P. falciparum malaria

1135
During the course of acute tubular necrosis
A pulmonary oedema is a recognised complication of the oliguric phase

B the elevated blood urea is the factor directly responsible for the majority of the clinical features

C the patient is more than usually susceptible to systemic infection

D the oliguric phase typically lasts for a month or more

E flaccid paralysis is a recognised complication during the diuretic phase

1136
In thyrotoxicosis
A there is a preponderance of females over males in the ratio of 8 : 1

B serum TSH levels are typically increased

C spontaneous remission is unknown

D toxic nodular goitres are commoner in older patients

E an IgG auto-antibody is the most probable explanation of the condition in a neonate

1137
The symptoms of phaeochromocytoma
A include sweating

B include flushing of the face as the most constant feature

C depend on the relative amounts of noradrenaline and adrenaline secreted

D may need urgent control by intravenous phentolamine

E may resemble those of acute anxiety

1138
At the menopause
A progesterone production is unimpaired

B depression may be severe enough to result in suicidal tendencies

C insomnia is a common troublesome symptom

D pruritus vulvae may be troublesome even in the absence of diabetes mellitus

E back pain and obesity occurring together are most often due to Cushing's syndrome

1139
Hypochromic anaemia in infants
A is easier to recognise clinically than in adults

B is unlikely to occur in those who are breast-fed

C occurs in premature babies because they have a small circulating red cell mass

D is not likely to be due to gluten-induced enteropathy since this does not usually appear till the age of 5

E bears no relation to the haematological status of the mother

1140
In a patient who suffers acute blood loss
A hypotension occurs after the sudden loss of one litre

B the rapid loss of 2–3 litres is usually fatal

C a reticulocytosis as high as 10 per cent may be expected during recovery

D the MCHC falls during convalescence even if iron supplies are adequate

E leucopenia is to be expected

1141
Parenteral iron therapy
A is suitable for patients with coeliac disease

B with iron-sorbitol is contra-indicated in renal failure

C with iron-dextran, unlike iron-sorbitol, should be given by the intravenous route

D should usually be combined with oral iron therapy

E is the treatment of choice for sideroblastic anaemia

1142
In a patient with myelomatosis
A Bence Jones protein consists of light chains of immunoglobulin

B a very rapid E.S.R. is suggestive of a super-added infection

C it is usual to find splenomegaly

D hypercalcaemia is an indication for treatment with corticosteroids

E amyloidosis may be responsible for renal failure

1143
In a haemorrhagic disorder
A the presence of urticaria suggests that acute nephritis may develop
B senile purpura occurs most commonly on the dorsum of the hand
C perifollicular haemorrhages on the legs suggest the possibility of scurvy
D hereditary haemorrhagic telangiectasia is a likely cause if the patient's mother was similarly affected
E petechiae are most profuse on the forehead and neck

1144
In a patient with a bleeding tendency
A treatment with heparin is sometimes indicated
B hypoprothrombinaemia is likely if the patient is less than three days old
C factor IX deficiency is a likely cause if the patient is a female
D the presence of spider telangiectases may be of diagnostic significance
E there may be excessive production of abnormal platelets

1145
The following statements about rheumatoid arthritis are correct:
A Aseptic necrosis of the head of the femur is a recognised feature
B Cervical spine involvement can lead to instability of the atlantoaxial articulation
C Temporomandibular involvement is common
D Muscular stiffness develops late while ankylosis is occurring
E Muscular atrophy in relation to affected joints is an early feature

1146
A male patient, aged 20, consults you because of episodes of unconsciousness. The following features support the idea that the attacks may be epileptic:
A Dimness or loss of vision for several seconds before the loss of consciousness
B Incontinence of urine during the attack
C Reports by observers of jerking movements during the attack
D Attacks provoked by flickering lights
E Attacks occurring after periods of prolonged standing

1147
Petit mal
A invariably starts in childhood
B is typically followed by a period of normal sleep
C may give place in adolescence to grand mal
D may persist into adult life
E gives rise to characteristic e.e.g. changes

1148
In a hemiplegic patient cerebral embolism as a cause would be favoured by
A a history of very abrupt onset
B the presence of a mitral diastolic murmur
C the finding of a haemoglobin of 18 gm/100 ml
D a blood pressure of 200/140 mm Hg
E the presence of a subhyaloid haemorrhage

1149
Disorganised joints (Charcot's) may be a consequence of
A multiple sclerosis
B tabes dorsalis
C motor neurone disease
D diabetes mellitus
E syringomyelia

1150
A clue to the aetiology of peripheral neuropathy may be given by the presence of
A glossitis
B haemoptysis
C similarly affected siblings
D eosinophilia
E Kayser-Fleischer rings

1151
Causes of transient cerebral ischaemic attacks include
A severe hypertension
B hypotension
C cervical spondylosis
D subclavian artery stenosis
E carotid artery stenosis

1152
A depressed patient
A with symptoms of disturbance of sleep, appetite and energy is best treated with a tricyclic antidepressant
B on tranylcypromine may well complain of difficulty with reading
C on phenelzine should be warned not to eat cheese
D with prolonged phobic symptoms is best treated with a mono-amine oxidase inhibitor
E on imipramine may well complain of difficulty in micturition

1153
Expected findings on investigation of a patient with tropical sprue include
A dimorphic anaemia
B hypoproteinaemia
C normal histological appearance of jejunal mucosa
D *Giardia intestinalis* in the stools
E spastic narrowing of the small intestine seen on barium meal and follow through

1154
Factors which may account for the high incidence of liver disease in tropical Africa include
A trypanosomiasis
B aflatoxin in ground nuts
C ancylostomiasis
D high prevalence of hepatitis B virus
E cyanide in cassava

1155
Anaemia due to glucose-6-phosphate dehydrogenase (G6PD) deficiency is typically precipitated by
A flying at high altitude
B the ingestion of broad beans (Vicia faba)
C treatment with antimalarials
D exposure to cold
E splenectomy

1156
In malaria due to *P. malariae*
A asymptomatic parasitaemia may persist for many years
B bouts of fever characteristically recur after 72 hours
C bouts consist of cold, hot and sweating stages in succession
D immune-complex nephritis is a recognised complication
E primaquine destroys the parasites both in the blood and in the liver

1157
Cholera
A infection by biotype El Tor has spread widely in recent years
B is notifiable under International Health Regulations
C is maintained between epidemics by a reservoir in rodents
D causes acute inflammation of the small intestine
E vibrios can be cultured from the blood during the early bacteraemic phase

1158
Dengue fever
A spreads by the faecal-oral route
B causes intense orbital and periarticular pain
C produces a rash during the second hump of the 'saddle-back' fever
D gives rise to a marked tachycardia, thought to be associated with myocarditis
E in its haemorrhagic form has a hospital mortality rate of up to 10 per cent in S.E. Asia

1159
In ancylostomiasis
A the larval stage takes place in the freshwater crustacean, *Cyclops*
B the larvae circulate to the lung and then penetrate into the alveoli
C the worms attach themselves to the small intestinal mucosa by their buccal capsules
D a heavy infection may result in an illness resembling kwashiorkor
E mass treatment of the entire population with piperazine salts is a valuable way of controlling the disease

1160
Infection by *Histoplasma capsulatum*
A is confined to North America
B is an occupational hazard for speleologists in an endemic area
C is confirmed by the presence of the parasites in a biopsied lymph node
D in the lungs may resemble primary or post-primary tuberculosis
E in its disseminated form resembles Hodgkin's disease

Section 2

In this section the questions are of the One-from-Five type, i.e. only *one* of the items is correct

M 1161

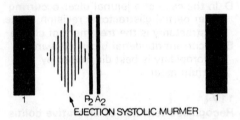

EJECTION SYSTOLIC MURMER

The ausculatory findings in the diagram above are compatible with a diagnosis of
A pulmonary stenosis
B mitral regurgitation
C ventricular septal defect
D aortic stenosis
E all of the above

M 1162

The least reliable way of identifying the dominant hemisphere of the brain is by asking the patient which
A hand he uses for writing
B hand he uses for cutting bread
C hand he uses to catch a ball
D foot he uses to kick a ball
E eye he would use for looking through a telescope

M 1163

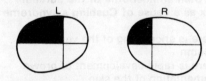

The visual field defect shown above is most likely to be caused by a lesion of
A the optic radiation
B the occipital cortex
C the optic chiasma
D the lateral geniculate body
E the optic tract

1164
The commonest autosomal recessive trait known in Western Europe is
A Friedreich's ataxia
B glycogen storage disease
C galactosaemia
D congenital adrenal hyperplasia
E none of the above

1165
Neutrophil polymorphonuclear leucocytosis is a characteristic feature of
A whooping-cough
B tuberculosis
C typhoid fever
D pneumococcal infection
E rubella

1166
Throughout the world the commonest cause of ill-health is
A malignant disease
B disease due to infection
C malnutrition
D degenerative arterial disease
E osteoarthrosis

1167
Neonates are particularly susceptible to
A scarlet fever
B measles
C whooping-cough
D rubella
E all of the above

1168
The total body water content of a 65 Kg man is approximately
A 24 litres
B 30 litres
C 40 litres
D 48 litres
E 52 litres

1169
The most common cause of acute circulatory failure (shock) is
A bacteraemia
B massive pulmonary embolism
C loss of fluid
D myocardial infarction
E paroxysmal tachycardia

1170
During pregnancy significant cardiac disease is suggested by
A increasing breathlessness between the 12th and 24th week
B tachycardia
C a fall in diastolic pressure
D displacement of the apex beat to the left
E a third heart sound

1171
Recognised complications of bronchial carcinoma include
A hoarseness
B superior vena caval obstruction
C lymphatic spread to the scalene nodes
D fits
E all of the above

1172

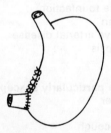

The operation illustrated above is a
A Billroth II partial gastrectomy
B gastroenterostomy
C Billroth I partial gastrectomy
D pyloroplasty
E Polya partial gastrectomy

1173
The following statements are correct:
A A gastro-jejuno-colic fistula is best demonstrated by barium meal
B Anastomotic (suture) ulcers are characteristically associated with a high acid output
C Biliary gastritis may symptomatically mimic gastric carcinoma
D In the case of a jejunal ulcer occurring after partial gastrectomy revision of the gastrectomy is the treatment of choice
E Recurrent duodenal ulcer following pyloroplasty is best diagnosed by barium meal

1174
Recognised features of ulcerative colitis include
A tenesmus
B colonic perforation
C constipation, when the disease is confined to the distal colon
D abnormal liver function tests
E all of the above

1175
In an elderly patient who complains of a recent change in bowel habit carcinoma is more likely than diverticular disease if there is
A rectal bleeding
B constipation alternating with diarrhoea
C pneumaturia
D a mass in the left iliac fossa
E marked weight loss

1176
An ectopic ACTH syndrome is more likely than an adenoma of the adrenal cortex as a cause of Cushing's syndrome if
A there is shortening of the vertebral column
B there is rapid development of brown pigmentation of the skin
C purple striae appear early
D diabetes mellitus is present
E there is virilisation in a female patient

1177
The following statements about rheumatoid arthritis are correct:
A In the early phase radiological examination reveals demineralisation of the bone ends
B The rheumatoid factor is usually an IgG antibody
C The Rose-Waaler test is diagnostically specific
D The joint fluid is of high viscosity
E Subcutaneous nodules appear in the majority of patients

1178
An acute attack of migraine can be relieved or aborted by the early administration of
A methysergide
B ergotamine tartrate
C diazepam
D reserpine
E tyramine

1179
Deep coma on admission to hospital of a poisoned patient is likely to be due to
A carbon monoxide
B salicylate
C morphine
D nitrazepam
E amphetamine

1180
For those travelling overland from Europe to S.E. Asia vaccinations required under International Health Regulations include
A typhoid and paratyphoid (TAB)
B smallpox
C yellow fever
D plague
E typhus

Section 3

The following questions are of the Relationship Analysis type and careful attention to the instructions is essential.

Each question consists of two statements linked by the word BECAUSE. The first statement is an assertion and the second an alleged reason for that assertion. The correct answer for each is one of the letters A to E according to the following key:

A Assertion and reason are true statements and the reason is a correct explanation of the assertion.
B Assertion and reason are true statements but the reason is not a correct explanation of the assertion.
C Assertion is true but reason is a false statement.
D Assertion is false but reason is a true statement.
E Both assertion and reason are false statements.

M 1181
At the outset of a clinical examination it is advisable for the doctor to appear to be pre-occupied with other matters BECAUSE a patient may take a few minutes to adapt himself to the situation.

M 1182
Examination of a baby for possible congenital hypertrophic pyloric stenosis is best carried out some hours after the last feed BECAUSE the pyloric tumour is difficult to feel during relaxation.

M 1183
In a child under the age of five who has suffered neurological damage, intelligence tests may be misleading BECAUSE the tests in children of this age depend largely on verbal skills.

M 1184
A deaf child usually exhibits poverty of gesture and movement BECAUSE the sensory deprivation of deafness causes a parallel lack of awareness of visual stimuli.

M 1185
In babies the passage of a fine polythene tube into the stomach through the mouth or nose for gastric juice samples is easy BECAUSE active swallowing is not necessary.

M 1186
Venepuncture is less satisfactory in babies than in older children BECAUSE an adequate amount of blood can usually be collected by heel puncture.

1187
Vasodilatation is a feature of beriberi BECAUSE autonomic nerves are affected in that disorder.

1188
Salt depletion rapidly reduces the volume of the extracellular fluid BECAUSE sodium is predominantly extracellular.

1189
The administration of carbonic anhydrase inhibitors causes potassium depletion BECAUSE these drugs increase the tubular secretion of hydrogen ions.

1190
Patients with bronchogenic carcinoma may show features of water intoxication BECAUSE such tumours may secrete a polypeptide with antidiuretic properties.

1191
Sodium retention is a recognised complication of chlorpropamide therapy BECAUSE chlorpropamide has an antidiuretic hormone-like effect.

1192
Benzothiadiazine diuretics depress the reabsorption of sodium in the distal convoluted tubule BECAUSE they inhibit carbonic anhydrase.

1193
In the treatment of pulmonary tuberculosis in children ethambutol is to be preferred to streptomycin BECAUSE the vestibular damage which streptomycin may cause is particularly disabling in this age group.

1194
In Gilbert's disease, there is a reduced ability to conjugate bilirubin BECAUSE there is a deficiency of glucuronyl transferase.

1195
In the Dubin-Johnson syndrome there is a rise in the serum concentration of unconjugated bilirubin BECAUSE there is a reduced ability to transport organic anions into the biliary canaliculi.

1196
Polyuria is a recognised feature of hyperparathyroidism BECAUSE there is, in this condition, an increased urinary excretion of calcium.

1197
Polyuria occurs during the recovery phase of acute renal failure BECAUSE secretion of vasopressin is diminished at this time.

1198
Osteosclerosis occurs in chronic glomerulonephritis BECAUSE the kidney is unable to convert dietary vitamin D to its active metabolite 1,25 dihydroxycholecalciferol in this condition.

1199
The Coomb's test is positive in hereditary spherocytosis BECAUSE the red cells do not assume their abnormal form unless an excess of antibody is present.

1200
In tropical Africa megaloblastic anaemia is more commonly due to folate than vitamin B_{12} deficiency BECAUSE the much smaller body store of folate is more vulnerable to depletion than the store of vitamin B_{12}.

Answers

PART ONE 1

Question	Answer	Question	Answer	Question	Answer	Question	Answer
1	AE	46	BCE	91	BDE	136	BCD
2	ABCE	47	BD	92	ABD	137	AC
3	ABCDE	48	BC	93	BC	138	ACDE
4	ACE	49	BDE	94	ABE	139	BCD
5	ACDE	50	ABDE	95	ACE	140	BCD
6	DE	51	ABC	96	ABD	141	E
7	AC	52	ACD	97	ACE	142	CE
8	CD	53	ABC	98	BD	143	B
9	ABD	54	ABDE	99	ABCE	144	ABCDE
10	AC	55	AE	100	AE	145	BC
11	BCD	56	BCE	101	BCDE	146	ABC
12	D	57	E	102	ACE	147	CD
13	CD	58	ACE	103	AD	148	AD
14	ACE	59	AE	104	BCE	149	ABDE
15	BDE	60	AC	105	ABCDE	150	ABE
16	A	61	DE	106	CDE	151	BCE
17	BC	62	CD	107	ABE	152	CE
18	BCE	63	BDE	108	BD	153	ABE
19	ACDE	64	CDE	109	BCD	154	AC
20	BC	65	CDE	110	ABC	155	ABC
21	BCE	66	BD	111	BE	156	ABCD
22	ABDE	67	BD	112	ABCE	157	ABCE
23	AE	68	ACDE	113	BDE	158	BDE
24	CD	69	E	114	BCD	159	BC
25	ABE	70	BD	115	ABC	160	ABD
26	AC	71	DE	116	ACDE	161	AC
27	BDE	72	A	117	ABE	162	C
28	BE	73	BDE	118	AB	163	ACE
29	ACD	74	ABD	119	CE	164	D
30	ABDE	75	ABD	120	AB	165	ACDE
31	ABD	76	ABE	121	BCDE	166	AC
32	DE	77	BE	122	BCDE	167	BDE
33	ABE	78	CD	123	BD	168	BCE
34	ABE	79	AD	124	BD	169	AD
35	ABCE	80	ABCD	125	ABCD	170	ACE
36	BD	81	BD	126	BD	171	ABDE
37	AE	82	D	127	ABCD	172	CD
38	AC	83	ABD	128	AD	173	ACE
39	BCDE	84	BD	129	BCE	174	ACE
40	AD	85	ACE	130	ACE	175	BCE
41	BCD	86	C	131	BCE	176	ADE
42	ADE	87	BDE	132	D	177	ACD
43	ABE	88	CDE	133	ABE	178	BCD
44	ABE	89	CD	134	CD	179	CDE
45	BE	90	DE	135	C	180	ABDE

Question	Answer	Question	Answer	Question	Answer	Question	Answer
181	ABD	236	ABCE	288	CD	343	BC
182	CD	237	AB	289	ABE	344	BE
183	ABD	238	ACDE	290	BDE	345	ABE
184	CD	239	AB	291	CD	346	BCDE
185	BDE	240	CE	292	BCE	347	BCE
186	BCDE	241	ACDE	293	CE	348	BCE
187	AE	242	ABD	294	BCD	349	ADE
188	BCDE	243	AD	295	BD	350	BC
189	BD	244	AB	296	ACE	351	CDE
190	CDE	245	ABD	297	BDE	352	BDE
191	BCD	246	ACE	298	BDE	353	BD
192	ACE	247	AB	299	ABC	354	BE
193	CD	248	ACD	300	ABC	355	BDE
194	All false	249	ABE	301	ABE	356	ACE
195	BDE	250	ADE	302	CDE	357	CDE
196	DE			303	ABE	358	ABE
197	ADE	**PART ONE 2**		304	ABD	359	AD
198	CD			305	ACD	360	D
199	ABE	251	ACD	306	BE	361	ABE
200	AB	252	CD	307	ABE	362	ADE
201	AE	253	ACE	308	ACE	363	ABCD
202	AE	254	ADE	309	BD	364	AC
203	AC	255	AC	310	ACDE	365	BDE
204	ACDE	256	ABE	311	BDE	366	ABE
205	BCDE	257	BCDE	312	BCDE	367	ACD
206	BCE	258	AC	313	ADE	368	ACD
207	ABC	259	BCE	314	DE	369	DE
208	ABCD	260	ABDE	315	ADE	370	ACE
209	ACE	261	AC	316	ABE	371	ACDE
210	BC	262	ABC	317	CE	372	DE
211	ABD	263	CDE	318	BCD	373	BCD
212	BD	264	BCD	319	BCE	374	ACD
213	BCDE	265	BCE	320	B	375	A
214	BCE	266	ACE	321	BD	376	ABD
215	ABCD	267	ADE	322	ACD	377	ACE
216	ABCDE	268	ACDE	323	B	378	BD
217	B	269	BCD	324	BDE	379	CDE
218	D	270	BCE	325	ABCE	380	ACDE
219	ABCDE	271	ACDE	326	AE	381	ABE
220	ACE	272	ADE	327	AD	382	BCD
221	ABE	273	BE	328	BCD	383	ABCD
222	BD	274	CD	329	CE	384	AD
223	BD	275	ACDE	330	ABD	385	ACD
224	BDE	276	ACE	331	ACDE	386	ABDE
225	ACE	277	ABC	332	BCE	387	ADE
226	BCE	278	AB	333	BCE	388	ACE
227	BD	279	BDE	334	ABCE	389	ACDE
228	BCDE	280	AB	335	ACE	390	AB
229	BDE	281	ABCE	336	BCD	391	BCD
230	ABD	282	ABE	337	BDE	392	AD
231	ABCD	283	AC	338	BE	393	ABCE
232	ACDE	284	ABE	339	ABCD	394	BCD
233	ABE	285	ABCE	340	BCE	395	ABDE
234	BCE	286	BCD	341	CDE	396	C
235	BCDE	287	BDE	342	ABDE	397	ABCE

Question	Answer	Question	Answer	Question	Answer	Question	Answer
398	BDE	453	BCD	508	ABD	563	BCD
399	AD	454	B	509	ABD	564	B
400	ABDE	455	ABC	510	DE	565	BCDE
401	BCDE	456	AC	511	ABCE	566	ABCDE
402	ACD	457	CD	512	AC	567	D
403	BCDE	458	ABCE	513	BCE	568	ACE
404	ABE	459	BCDE	514	CDE	569	AD
405	BC	460	AB	515	BCDE	570	B
406	ABD	461	ABCDE	516	ABE	571	CD
407	CE	462	ACD	517	BD	572	ABE
408	BE	463	AE	518	BCD	573	ABE
409	BC	464	ACD	519	BCDE	574	B
410	BE	465	E	520	BDE	575	CD
411	BCD	466	ACDE	521	ACD	576	ABCDE
412	ABE	467	BCDE	522	ACD	577	BCD
413	ABCDE	468	DE	523	BDE	578	AD
414	ABD	469	AC	524	ACD	579	E
415	BCDE	470	ABCD	525	ABE	580	BCDE
416	ACD	471	CE	526	BCDE	581	D
417	BE	472	ADE	527	AC	582	BE
418	CD	473	ACDE	528	BD	583	ABCDE
419	BC	474	BCD	529	BCD	584	BC
420	BE	475	AD	530	ABE	585	BCE
421	ADE	476	AC	531	BE	586	BD
422	BE	477	BE	532	ABDE	587	CDE
423	B	478	DE	533	BCD	588	A
424	AD	479	ABD	534	DE	589	AD
425	AE	480	BCDE	535	BE	590	ACD
426	ACE	481	ACE	536	BCE	591	CE
427	BCDE	482	DE	537	ACD	592	ABD
428	ACD	483	ABCE	538	BCD	593	BE
429	ADE	484	ACE	539	BDE	594	BD
430	BCE	485	ACD	540	CE	595	CE
431	AE	486	CE	541	DE	596	CD
432	BD	487	ABE	542	All false	597	ABDE
433	BCD	488	ABC	543	ABC	598	B
434	AB	489	ACD	544	ABD	599	DE
435	ABDE	490	BCD	545	ADE	600	ABCDE
436	D	491	ACD	546	CE	601	BE
437	ABC	492	ABCD	547	B	602	BCDE
438	D	493	BE	548	CE	603	ACD
439	ADE	494	BDE	549	BCE	604	AE
440	D	495	BC	550	ABDE	605	AC
441	AE	496	CD	551	CDE	606	ABC
442	CD	497	ACE	552	ABCDE	607	ACE
443	BD	498	ABCD	553	BCE	608	ADE
444	D	499	ACD	554	ABD	609	AE
445	ABD	500	AD	555	D	610	BCE
446	ABE	501	BE	556	ABC	611	CDE
447	BCD	502	BCD	557	C	612	ABDE
448	ACE	503	AB	558	CD	613	CE
449	BCD	504	BC	559	CD	614	ABC
450	E	505	ABDE	560	ABCD	615	BD
451	DE	506	BCD	561	ACE	616	CDE
452	ADE	507	ABE	562	CDE	617	ABCD

Question	Answer	Question	Answer	Question	Answer	Question	Answer
618	BD	673	ACD	728	E	783	ACE
619	CDE	674	ABD	729	AC	784	CDE
620	ABC	675	BE	730	CDE	785	BCE
621	BE	676	ABCDE	731	ACD	786	ACD
622	All false	677	CD	732	ABC	787	ACDE
623	BCDE	678	DE	733	BCDE	788	C
624	BD	679	BC	734	DE	789	BCD
625	ADE	680	BDE	735	BE	790	BCD
626	ABCD	681	CD	736	ADE	791	ACE
627	B	682	ACD	737	ABCE	792	BC
628	ACD	683	CD	738	D	793	ACDE
629	ABC	684	ACD	739	ACE	794	CE
630	ABDE	685	BD	740	BCE	795	AC
631	BC	686	ACDE	741	BCD	796	ABD
632	ACE	687	ACD	742	BCDE	797	CDE
633	BDE	688	BD	743	CD	798	BCD
634	ABDE	689	CD	744	CD	799	ABD
635	BDE	690	ABCDE	745	BCD	800	AB
636	B	691	AD	746	CD	801	BDE
637	BCE	692	BCD	747	BDE	802	BCDE
638	ABD	693	ABCE	748	ABCD	803	BD
639	BCD	694	AE	749	AE	804	ABCE
640	ABD	695	ACDE	750	BCE	805	ABDE
641	A	696	ADE	751	BDE	806	ABE
642	CD	697	CE	752	ACDE	807	ACE
643	DE	698	CE	753	CE	808	AD
644	All false	699	ACE	754	CD	809	ABCDE
645	ADE	700	ABCD	755	ABCDE	810	ABCE
646	AC	701	ABC	756	BDE	811	DE
647	ABCDE	702	ACDE	757	BDE	812	BC
648	CDE	703	ABCDE	758	BCDE	813	ABD
649	D	704	ACE	759	BD	814	ACE
650	AB	705	BCD	760	AC	815	ABCE
651	ACE	706	BCDE	761	AC	816	ABCE
652	A	707	D	762	ABCE	817	DE
653	ADE	708	D	763	E	818	ABD
654	BDE	709	BCD	764	ABD	819	CE
655	A	710	BDE	765	ACE	820	A
656	AD	711	BD	766	BDE	821	BDE
657	ACD	712	CD	767	CDE	822	DE
658	D	713	ABCDE	768	ABDE	823	ACD
659	ABCE	714	BDE	769	BE	824	CE
660	ABC	715	DE	770	ACD	825	ACE
661	E	716	BCD	771	CDE	826	ABC
662	BCD	717	BD	772	ABDE	827	BCD
663	ABDE	718	CDE	773	ABC	828	CDE
664	ABE	719	BE	774	ACE	829	AD
665	CE	720	ABD	775	AE	830	ABCE
666	ACE	721	ABD	776	BDE	831	ADE
667	AE	722	ACDE	777	AB	832	BCD
668	A	723	BDE	778	AC	833	BC
669	A	724	ABCE	779	ACD	834	ACD
670	CD	725	BC	780	C	835	ACDE
671	ACE	726	BD	781	BD	836	ABCE
672	AE	727	A	782	ABCD	837	B

Question	Answer	Question	Answer	Question	Answer	Question	Answer
838	ABE	893	AC	948	ABCD	1003	AC
839	BCDE	894	ABCD	949	BD	1004	BCD
840	BCD	895	ABCD	950	ACD	1005	E
841	ABC	896	BDE	951	BCDE	1006	CE
842	BDE	897	CDE	952	ADE	1007	ABCE
843	AB	898	ABCD	953	DE	1008	CD
844	BE	899	ABC	954	C	1009	ACD
845	ABE	900	BC	955	CDE	1010	ACE
846	B	901	ABD	956	ABD	1011	CD
847	BD	902	ABDE	957	ABDE	1012	ADE
848	BDE	903	AC	958	AD	1013	CD
849	ACD	904	ABCD	959	BC	1014	C
850	ABE	905	ABCE	960	BCE	1015	BCD
851	BC	906	ACE	961	AB	1016	D
852	CD	907	BCE	962	ACDE	1017	ADE
853	ACE	908	ACDE	963	ACE	1018	D
854	BCE	909	BCE	964	ACE	1019	BE
855	C	910	CD	965	CDE	1020	ACD
856	CD	911	ACD	966	BD	1021	CDE
857	ABCE	912	ACDE	967	AC	1022	BE
858	CDE	913	ABCE	968	ACE	1023	ACE
859	ABCD	914	BC	969	BCD	1024	ACDE
860	ADE	915	ACDE	970	ABD	1025	ACD
861	ACDE	916	BCD	971	CE	1026	ABD
862	ADE	917	ADE	972	AB	1027	AD
863	ADE	918	BDE	973	AE	1028	ABCDE
864	ABCE	919	ABCE	974	BCE	1029	BCE
865	AD	920	DE	975	BCD	1030	ACD
866	ABCE	921	ABCD	976	BD	1031	BD
867	BDE	922	BC	977	ABCE	1032	BD
868	BDE	923	ABD	978	CDE	1033	ABD
869	BDE	924	ACD	979	ABCE	1034	AC
870	AE	925	BDE	980	CDE	1035	ADE
871	ACD	926	ABCDE	981	AC	1036	ABD
872	BDE	927	BDE	982	BD	1037	ACD
873	BC	928	AC	983	ACE	1038	AE
874	ABCD	929	AB	984	BCDE	1039	CDE
875	BCD	930	BCDE	985	CDE	1040	BD
876	ABDE	931	ABDE	986	ACE	1041	CDE
877	ACE	932	CDE	987	BCDE	1042	BD
878	ABD	933	ACD	988	BDE	1043	CDE
879	BDE	934	BCD	989	ADE	1044	AB
880	ABD	935	ACE	990	CD	1045	BE
881	ACE	936	ABCD	991	BCE	1046	ACD
882	ACD	937	BCE	992	ABC	1047	ACDE
883	BC	938	AE	993	ABDE	1048	ADE
884	ABC	939	ACE	994	AD	1049	ACE
885	BC	940	ADE	995	BC	1050	CDE
886	AB	941	CD	996	ABC	1051	ADE
887	CD	942	ADE	997	ABCD	1052	ACDE
888	BCDE	943	D	998	BDE	1053	BCE
889	ABDE	944	ABCE	999	BCE	1054	BDE
890	ABCD	945	ACE	1000	ABCE	1055	AE
891	ABC	946	ABC	1001	CD	1056	DE
892	ABCD	947	AB	1002	BC	1057	BC

Question	Answer	Question	Answer	Question	Answer	Question	Answer
1058	CD	1096	ABCDE	1131	ABD	1166	B
1059	ABDE	1097	BCE	1132	C	1167	C
1060	ACD	1098	CD	1133	ABCE	1168	C
1061	D	1099	ABE	1134	ABCD	1169	C
1062	ADE	1100	BC	1135	ACE	1170	A
1063	ABE			1136	ADE	1171	E
1064	BCE	**PART TWO 1**		1137	ACDE	1172	C
1065	C			1138	BCD	1173	C
1066	BD	1101	DE	1139	C	1174	E
1067	DE	1102	BCDE	1140	ABC	1175	E
1068	ABDE	1103	ABE	1141	ABC	1176	B
1069	BC	1104	BDE	1142	ADE	1177	A
1070	CD	1105	CE	1143	ABCD	1178	B
1071	ABCE	1106	BCE	1144	ABDE	1179	C
1072	CE	1107	ADE	1145	BE	1180	B
1073	ABD	1108	ABE	1146	BCD		
1074	AC	1109	AC	1147	ACDE	**PART TWO 3**	
1075	CE	1110	A	1148	AB		
1076	ADE	1111	AB	1149	BDE	1181	D
1077	ABD	1112	ACDE	1150	ABCD	1182	D
1078	BCD	1113	ACE	1151	ABCDE	1183	C
1079	ACD	1114	ABDE	1152	ACDE	1184	E
1080	CE	1115	AC	1153	AB	1185	A
1081	ACD	1116	D	1154	ABD	1186	B
1082	BDE	1117	AC	1155	BC	1187	B
1083	B	1118	BDE	1156	ABCD	1188	A
1084	C	1119	ADE	1157	AB	1189	C
1085	BE	1120	BDE	1158	BCE	1190	A
1086	ACE	1121	ACE	1159	BCD	1191	D
1087	CD	1122	AE	1160	BCDE	1192	B
1088	ABCD	1123	ABE			1193	E
1089	ABE	1124	ABE	**PART TWO 2**		1194	A
1090	ABE	1125	DE			1195	D
1091	BC	1126	BDE	1161	D	1196	B
1092	ABDE	1127	CDE	1162	A	1197	C
1093	CDE	1128	CE	1163	A	1198	B
1094	ABD	1129	ABD	1164	E	1199	E
1095	All false	1130	ABC	1165	D	1200	A